Guide to Home-Based Cancer Care: Chemotherapy & Radiotherapy

Editors-in-Chief: Liu Yan, Chen Yuanjiao

Translated by Weng Guizhen, Xu Shaoyuan

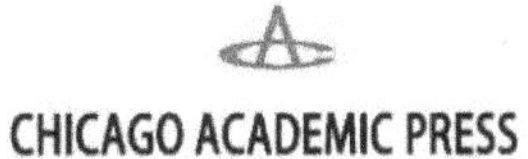

CHICAGO ACADEMIC PRESS

Guide to Home-Based Cancer Care: Chemotherapy & Radiotherapy
Editors-in-Chief: Liu Yan, Chen Yuanjiao
Translators: Weng Guizhen and Xu Shaoyuan
Language: English
Word Count (for the space of all pages): 203 Thousand Words
Publisher: Chicago Academic Press
Number of Pages: 314
ISBN: 978-1-965890-94-3

Publishing   Chicago Academic Press

                  5923 N Artesian Ave

                  Chicago IL 60659

Email   contact@chicagoacademicpress.com

Website   http://chicagoacademicpress.com/

Book Size   6X9 inches

First Edition   November, 2025

Personal Profile

Weng Guizhen, female, Master of Medicine, Deputy Chief Nurse, Tutor for postgraduate students, Head Nurse of the Department of Oncology, Fujian Medical University Union Hospital, National Certified Psychological Counselor (Level 2), and National Certified Public Nutritionist (Level 2). She is a member of the Review Expert Database for Fujian Provincial Standardized Treatment Demonstration Ward for Cancer Pain and Fujian Provincial Standardized Management Demonstration Ward for chemotherapy-induced nausea and vomiting (CINV), Head of the Pain Specialized Nursing Group, and Deputy Head of the Intravenous Therapy Specialized Nursing Group of Fujian Medical University Union Hospital. She has been committed to oncology clinical nursing and management for 16 years. She has presided over or participated in multiple Provincial/Bureau-level Research Projects, participated in multiple domestic and foreign oncology clinical trial research, published more than 10 articles as the first author or corresponding author, and participated in compiling 4 works. She concurrently serves as a member of the Palliative Care Professional Committee of the Ninth Council of Fujian Nursing Association, a standing member of the First Oncology Nursing Professional Committee of Fujian Anti-Cancer Association, a member of the First Oncology Psychology Professional Committee of Fujian Anti-Cancer Society, a member of the

Eighth Nursing Psychology Professional Collaboration Group of Fujian Mental Health Association, a member of the Third Committee of the Cross-Strait Medical Development Committee of Cross-Strait Medical and Health Exchange Association, and a director of the Oncology Nutrition Branch of Fujian Cross-Strait Medical and Health Exchange Association. She has extensive clinical experience in comprehensive oncology treatment nursing, cancer pain, and vascular access nursing.

Author's Affiliation:

1. Department of Oncology Nursing, Fujian Medical University Union Hospital, Fuzhou, Fujian, China.

2. School of Nursing, Fujian Medical University, Fuzhou, Fujian, China.

Xu Shaoyuan, female, Master of Medicine, Nurse-in-Charge, Head Nurse of the Department of Oncology, Fujian Maternity and Child Health Hospital, and National Certified Psychological Counselor (Level 2). From January 2024 to January 2025, she was a Visiting Scholar at the Waikato Institute of Technology in New Zealand. She holds several professional roles, including Youth Committee Member of the Oncology Nursing Professional Committee of the Chinese Nursing Association, Committee Member of the Oncology Nursing Professional Committee of the Fujian Nursing

Association, Oncology Specialized Nurse of the Fujian Nursing Association, and Bone Marrow Transplantation Specialized Nurse.

With nearly 17 years of experience in oncology nursing and nursing management, she has extensive expertise in clinical oncology nursing and administrative leadership. Her research focuses on oncology nursing and gynecological nursing. She has presided over one provincial-level Natural Science Fund project and has led multiple university- and hospital-level research projects. As first author, she has published seven papers included in SCI and CSCD databases and contributed to two monographs.

Author's Affiliation:

1. Department of Nursing, Fujian Maternity and Child Health Hospital College of Clinical Medicine for Obstetrics & Gynecology and Pediatrics, Fujian Medical University, Fuzhou City, Fujian Province, China.

2. School of Nursing, Fujian Medical University, Fuzhou City, Fujian Province, China.

Contents

Part 4: What to Eat During Chemotherapy?..................49

Part 1: What is Chemotherapy?

1. What is chemotherapy?

Chemotherapy refers to the use of chemical drugs to treat cancer by inhibiting cancer cell growth and preventing metastasis, ultimately aiming to control the disease.

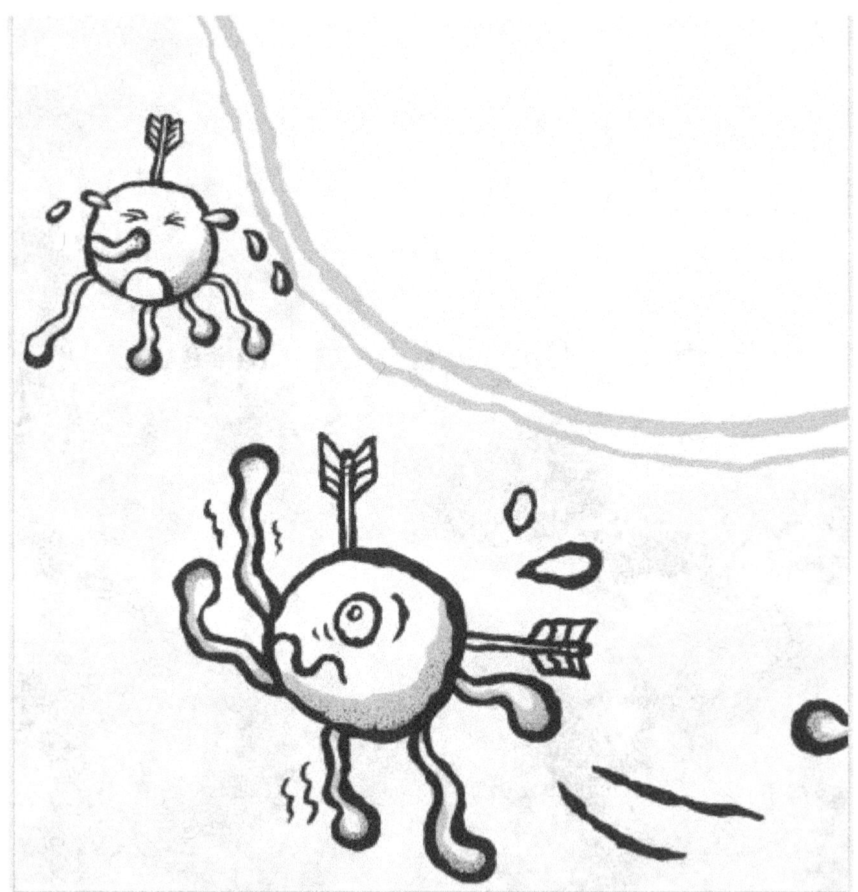

Chemotherapy, surgery, and radiotherapy are known as the three major treatments for cancer.

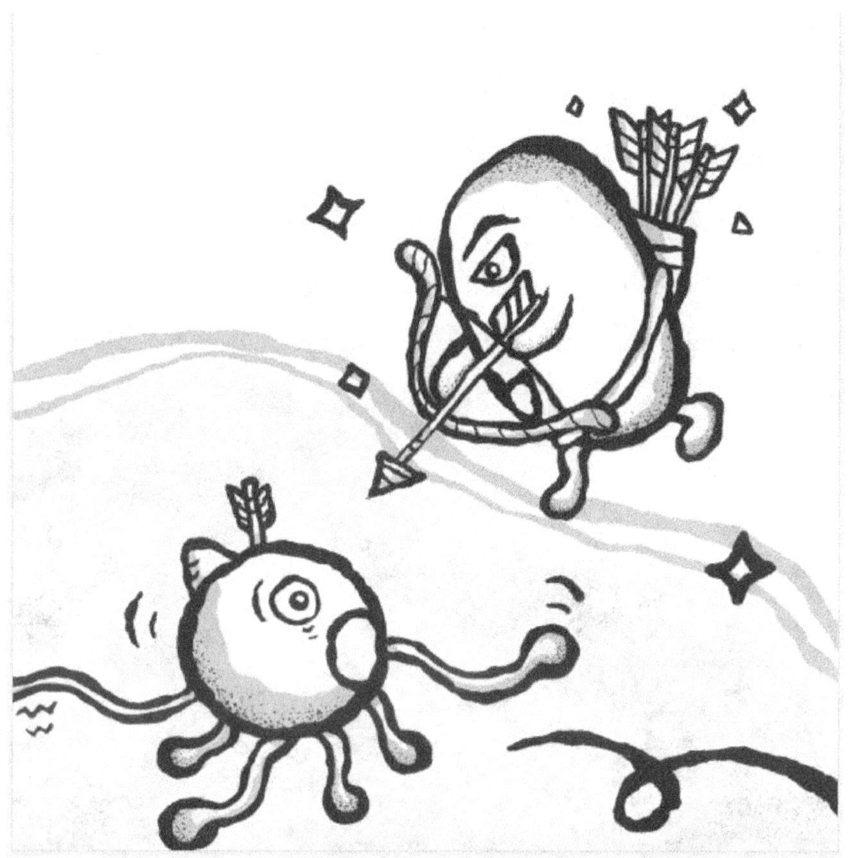

2. Why should patients undergo chemotherapy?

When patients have cancer, malignant cells in their bodies divide and spread uncontrollably, consuming essential nutrients. Chemotherapy can effectively shrink tumors while they are still small, making it a critical treatment for cancer. By reducing the number of cancerous cells, chemotherapy helps control tumor growth and progression. During treatment, the drugs circulate through the bloodstream, reaching affected tissues and organs. For this reason, chemotherapy is commonly used for patients with advanced or metastatic cancer, even when the disease has spread to other parts of the body.

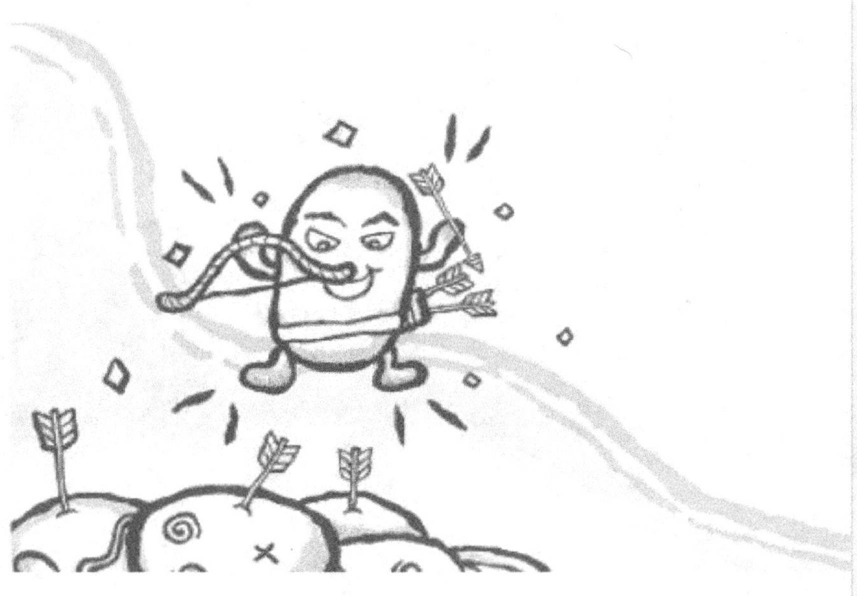

Cancer remains one of the most challenging diseases to overcome. While only a small percentage of patients can be cured by chemotherapy alone, there is no doubt that it can significantly extend survival and improve quality of life.

3. Chemotherapy category

1. Radical chemotherapy

Certain cancers that are highly responsive to chemotherapy—such as leukemia, lymphoma, choriocarcinoma, and germ cell tumors—can be cured with chemotherapy alone. When chemotherapy is administered with curative intent, it is referred to as Radical chemotherapy.

2. Palliative chemotherapy

In most cases of advanced cancer, where cancer cells have already metastasized widely, current technology makes a cure impossible. The purpose of chemotherapy is mainly to control the development of cancer to prolong patients' lives, or to improve their quality of life through chemotherapy. This type of chemotherapy is called palliative chemotherapy.

3. Postoperative adjuvant chemotherapy

Even after surgical removal of the tumor, undetectable micrometastases may have already occurred prior to surgery, or residual cancer cells may remain near the surgical site. Adjuvant chemotherapy is administered to eliminate these remaining cancer cells, thereby reducing the risk of recurrence and metastatic spread.

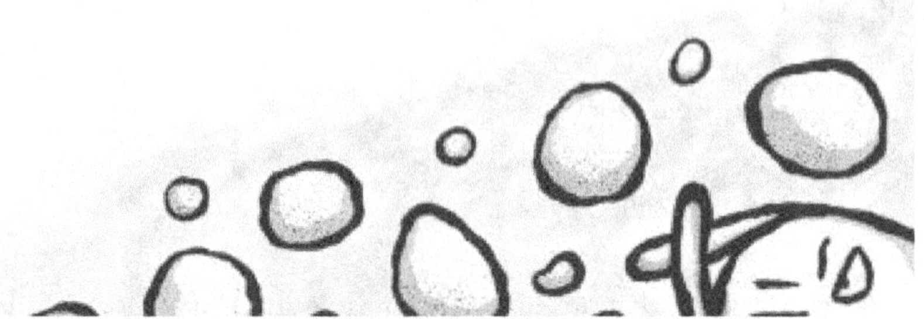

4. Preoperative chemotherapy (neoadjuvant chemotherapy)

Preoperative chemotherapy can shrink the lesions, making surgical resection easier, or shrink some lesions that have lost the chance of surgery so that they can be resected. It can also kill potential metastatic lesions and reduce the possibility of recurrence and metastasis.

5. Intracavitary chemotherapy

Administration of drugs into body cavities (e.g., intraperitoneal or intrathoracic) allows for temporarily elevated local drug concentrations, thereby enhancing therapeutic efficacy in the target region.

4. Methods of administration in chemotherapy

1. Intravenous administration

Intravenous administration is the most common method for delivering anticancer drugs. It is absorbed quickly and completely, but it has a local irritation effect. It is necessary to try to avoid phlebitis and drug leakage into the subcutaneous tissue, which may cause local tissue ulcers, necrosis, etc. In clinical practice, patients often use central venous catheters for medication. Before chemotherapy, patients have peripherally inserted central venous catheters (PICC), central venous catheters (CVC), or fully implantable infusion ports (PORT) in place in advance.

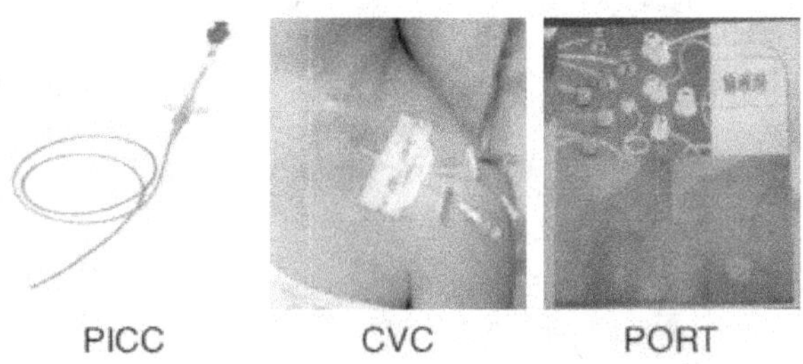

PICC   CVC   PORT

2. Oral administration

Oral administration typically causes fewer toxic side effects but may irritate the gastrointestinal tract, resulting in nausea, vomiting, or diarrhea. To minimize gastric mucosal irritation and protect the drug from stomach acid degradation, it is typically formulated in capsules or enteric-coated tablets. Common oral chemotherapy drugs include cyclohexylnitrosourea and capecitabine.

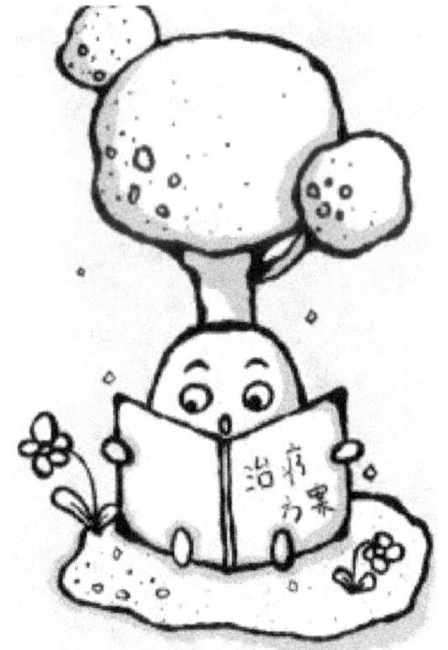

3. Intramuscular injection

Intramuscular injection offers better absorption than oral administration. This method is suitable for non-irritating drugs, such as bleomycin (BLM). Administering the injection deeply into the muscle enhances drug absorption. However, oil-based preparations like testosterone propionate have slower absorption rates, so it is essential to ensure deep intramuscular injection and alternating injection sites to avoid complications.

4. Intracavitary chemotherapy

Including intrathoracic chemotherapy, intraperitoneal chemotherapy, and intrapericardial chemotherapy. The characteristics of the drugs are: reusable, less local irritation, and good anti-cancer activity, such as mitomycin, cisplatin (DDP), etc.

5. Intra-arterial chemotherapy administration

For brain metastases of malignant tumors, anticancer drugs are

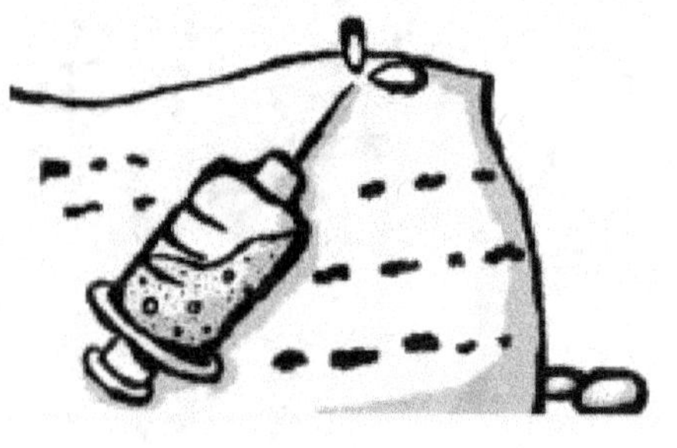

delivered via direct carotid artery injection. For malignant soft tissue tumors in the lower limbs, intra-arterial chemother -apy is administered through femoral artery puncture. In cases of unresectable malignancies—such as liver cancer—anticancer drugs may be infused directly into the exposed hepatic artery during surgery.

6. Intrathecal chemotherapy administration

Intrathecal chemotherapy drugs can be administered via lumbar puncture. The distribution of the drug can be significantly improved by lying down for a period of time after the injection.

7. Intratumoral injection

Local injection for cervical cancer and intravesical instillation for bladder cancer.

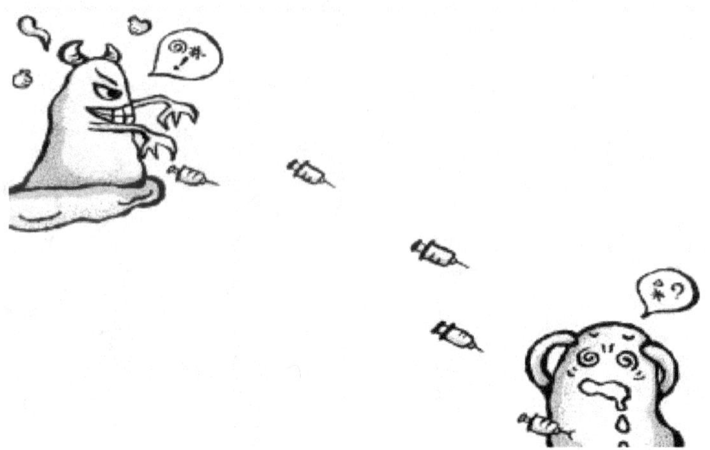

5. Indications for chemotherapy

The oncologist should determine the specific situation of patients. Chemotherapy should be given in the following situations:

(1) Malignant tumors that are sensitive to chemotherapy and are treated

with chemotherapy as the main treatment method may be cured through standardized chemotherapy. For example, small cell lung cancer, leukemia, malignant lymphoma, choriocarcinoma, germ cell malignant tumors, etc.

(2) For sensitive or relatively sensitive malignant tumors, chemotherapy should be performed before or after surgery.

(3) Palliative chemotherapy for advanced malignant tumors.

6. Contraindications to chemotherapy

(1) Patients whose physical condition is too poor or too old to tolerate chemotherapy.

(2) Those with severe organ dysfunction (such as severe liver and kidney dysfunction, etc.).

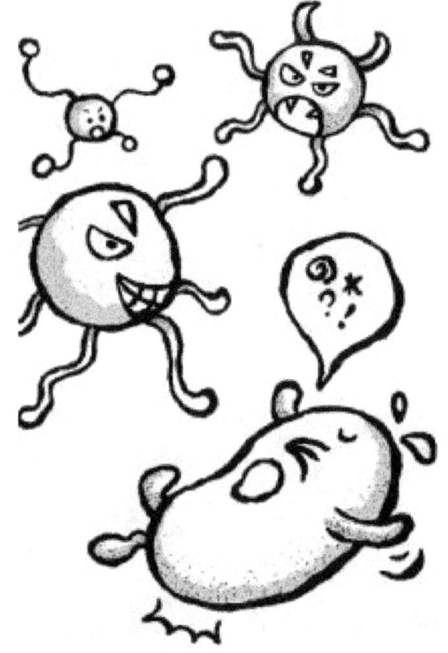

(3) Chemotherapy is generally not required for early-stage cancers (such as carcinoma in situ and stage I cancer) that have been successfully surgically removed.

(4) For patients who develop drug resistance after multiple rounds of chemotherapy and whose chemotherapy regimen is still ineffective, other

treatment methods should be chosen.

(5) Some cancers show minimal sensitivity to chemotherapy drugs, making it unlikely to achieve the desired therapeutic outcomes. In these cases, alternative treatments—such as biologic immunotherapy—may offer greater clinical benefit to patients.

Part 2: What to Prepare for Chemotherapy?

1. Chemotherapy tips

(1) Psychological: Prior to initiating chemotherapy, patients should be educated about potential treatment reactions and management strategies. This helps alleviate anxiety and psychological distress related to side effects while fostering confidence in overcoming the disease. Close collaboration with healthcare providers will help patients successfully complete their treatment course.

(2) Diet: Choose light, easily digestible, high-calorie, vitamin-rich foods, and eat more fresh vegetables and fruits. Pay attention to the color, aroma, and taste of food, and change the variety and type frequently to increase appetite. Avoid eating irritating foods, drinking alcohol, and drinking less coffee. After chemotherapy, drink more warm water to promote the excretion of the metabolites of chemotherapy drugs through urine and reduce their toxic side effects.

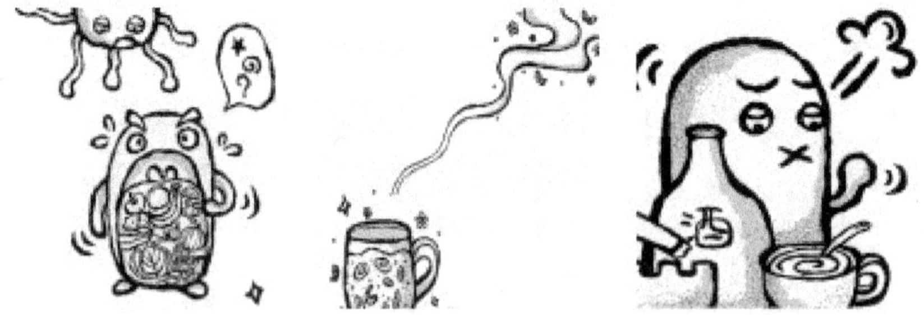

(3) Preparation before chemotherapy: Before chemotherapy, the heart, lung, liver, and kidney functions should be evaluated, and blood routine,

coagulation function, and electrocardiogram should be checked. If the white blood cell count is lower than 4.0×10^9/L, the body temperature exceeds the normal range, or patients have a cold, chemotherapy should not be performed. Female patients should avoid the menstrual period as much as possible. Before chemotherapy, diphenhydramine, dexamethasone, grenadetron hydrochloride, and other drugs should be given according to doctors' advice to prevent gastrointestinal reactions and allergic reactions.

(4) Life: Take good rest and get enough sleep. During chemotherapy, patients should prevent infection, avoid crowded places, avoid colds, ventilate the room frequently, keep the air fresh, and reduce the chance of contracting external infectious diseases. Pay attention to personal hygiene and keep hands clean. Monitor changes in body temperature, detect signs of infection early, and notify medical staff in time if there are any abnormalities.

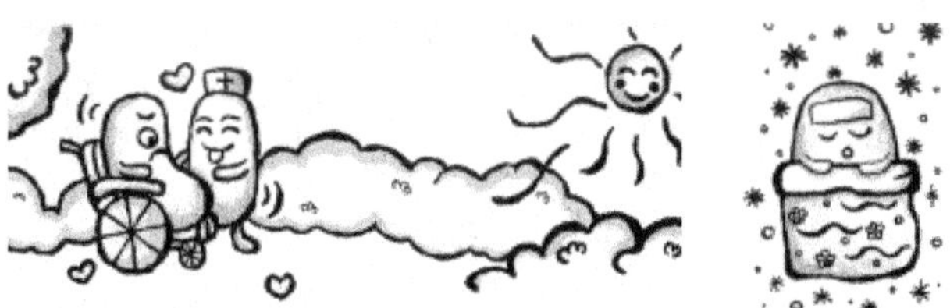

(5) Infusion guidance: Do not perform intravenous infusion on the surgical side. The limb receiving the infusion should not be moved too much

to prevent the puncture needle from moving, causing drug extravasation and local tissue necrosis. Do not apply hot compresses to the intravenous infusion site. Understand the precautions in drug use, focusing on how to protect blood vessels and prevent complications.

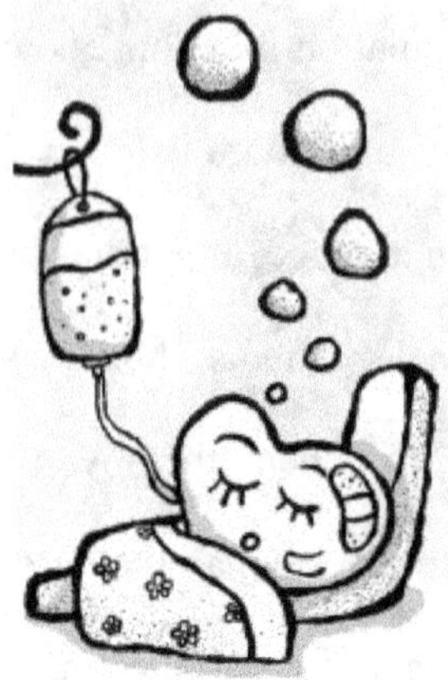

2. Preparation for chemotherapy

1. Before chemotherapy

(1) Complete various examinations, such as blood routine examination, liver and kidney function, cardiopulmonary function testing, etc.

(2) Pay attention to oral hygiene, develop good oral hygiene habits, and cut nails frequently.

(3) Since chemotherapy drugs have a strong irritating and corrosive effect on peripheral blood vessels, which can easily cause phlebitis and extravasation, it is recommended to place a central venous catheter during the first chemotherapy.

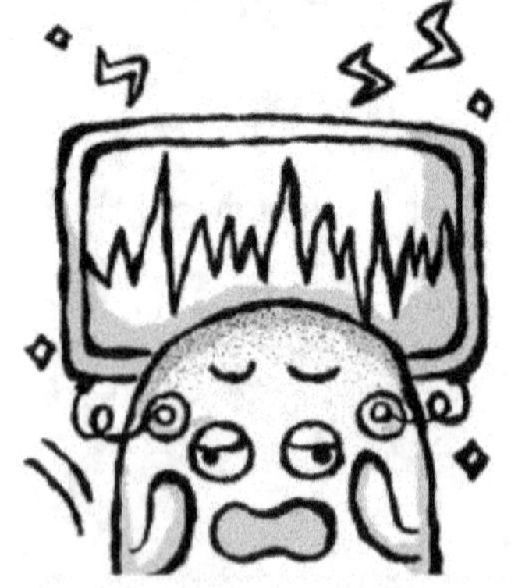

(4) Ensure adequate rest before chemotherapy and be fully prepared mentally.

2. During chemotherapy

(1) Remain as still as possible during chemotherapy administration. Immediately notify your nurse if you experience pain or any discomfort at the puncture site.

(2) Eat small meals frequently and diversify patients' diet. If vomiting occurs, eat during the intervals between vomiting.

(3) Keep the oral cavity clean and moist. If oral ulcers have occurred, take medication as prescribed by doctors. If there is large-scale oral and esophagitis, patients should temporarily fast.

(4) Drink plenty of water. The daily water intake should be more than 3000 mL, and the urine volume should be kept above 2000 mL.

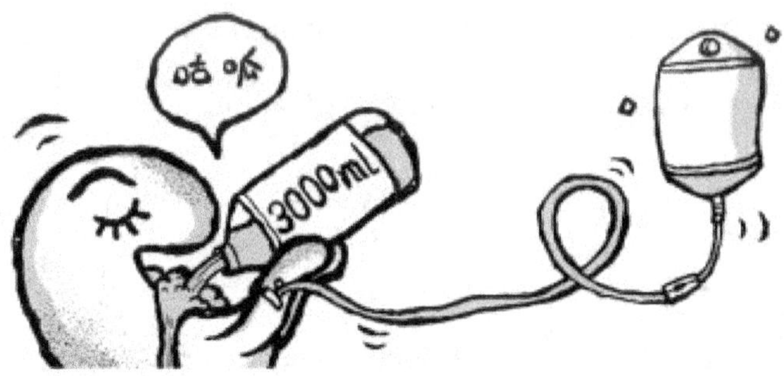

(5) During the infusion of methotrexate (MTX), pay attention to reducing the intake of highly acidic foods and maintaining the urine pH value between 7 and 8. Rinse the mouth as directed by the doctor to reduce the occurrence of oral ulcers.

(6) During the infusion of ifosfamide (IFO, Holusheng), avoid eating grapefruit or drinking grapefruit juice to avoid weakening the treatment effect.

(7) Do not be exposed to cold stimulation within 5 days of cisplatin (DDP) administration, such as avoiding outdoor activities in cold climates, not eating cold food, not drinking cold drinks, not touching cold surfaces or objects, not washing hands with cold water, and avoiding approaching air conditioners and refrigerators.

(8) During the use of etoposide (VP16), postural hypotension is likely to occur, so patients should change their posture slowly. If they experience symptoms such as dizziness, they should avoid getting out of bed. Keep the ward clean and tidy, and place items in order to prevent patients from getting hurt.

(9) Patients need to be accompanied by someone when getting out of bed, taking a bath, or going to the toilet to avoid falling.

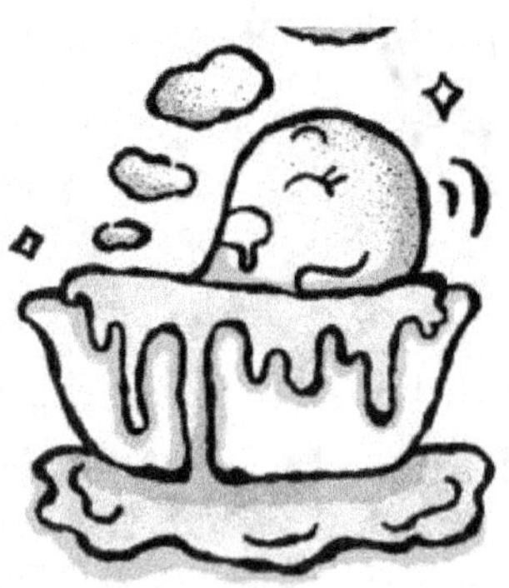

(10) When patients' white blood cell count is lower than 4.0×10^9/L, pay attention to changes in body temperature, wear a mask, avoid going to crowded places, reduce accompanying and visiting in the ward, and irradiate the room with ultraviolet light every day. When patients' white blood cell count is lower than 1.0×10^9/L, avoid eating raw and cold

food. All food must be heated before eating. The fruit eaten must be fresh and complete, without damage or insect bites, and must be cooked before eating. Drink warm water to avoid infection.

(11) If patients' platelet count is less than 100×10^9/L, care should be taken to prevent injuries during activities. Do not blow the nose forcefully. If nose bleeding occurs, notify medical staff immediately. Avoid emotional agitation, and children should avoid crying. Keep bowel movements open to prevent intracranial hemorrhage.

(12) When vomiting, patients should sit up or lie flat with the head tilted to one side to avoid dangerous aspiration of vomitus into the trachea.

(13) Do not adjust the infusion speed at will during the infusion to avoid causing unnecessary harm to patients. If patients have any questions, contact the nurse on duty in a timely manner.

(14) Keep warm and avoid catching a cold.

3. After intravenous chemotherapy

(1) After the injection, the nurse will check again and doctors will remind patients to avoid colds and infections, because chemotherapy will weaken the body's immune system and make patients more susceptible to infection.

(2) Patients are generally advised to maintain adequate hydration for 48 hours following chemotherapy to facilitate drug metabolism and elimination.

(3) After chemotherapy, be sure to remove all body fluids and waste, because the drugs will remain in the body for about 48 hours after treatment, which may affect family members. Body fluids and excretions include: urine, defecation, vomitus, and genital-related fluids.

(4) After chemotherapy, get more rest, drink plenty of water, try to keep a calm and happy mood, maintain an optimistic and cheerful attitude, face reality bravely, overcome the physical discomfort caused by chemotherapy, and insist on receiving chemotherapy.

(5) Maintain a regular lifestyle, quit smoking and drinking, master a correct and reasonable diet, drink plenty of water, and avoid spicy, greasy, and other irritating foods.

(6) Keep the mouth clean, brush the teeth with warm water and a soft-bristled toothbrush, arrange daily life reasonably, get more rest, avoid overwork, and try to avoid crowded public places to prevent infection.

(7) Regularly check blood routine, liver, and kidney function to detect abnormalities early and seek medical attention promptly.

4. During chemotherapy and 48 hours after

(1) Flush the toilet twice after each use to reduce residual drug exposure.

Close the toilet lid before flushing to minimize splashing. If possible, use a separate toilet during this time. If this is not possible, wear disposable gloves to clean the toilet seat after each use. Both male and female patients should sit on the toilet when using the toilet. This helps to reduce splashing. After using the toilet, wash hands with warm water and soap. Dry hands with a paper towel.

When vomiting into a toilet, be sure to clean up any splashes and flush the toilet twice. When vomiting into a bucket or basin, carefully pour it into the toilet without splashing, then flush it twice. Clean the bucket or basin with hot, soapy water, rinse it, pour the rinse water into the toilet, and then flush. Dry the bucket or basin with a paper towel and throw the paper towel away.

(2) If a caregiver needs to touch patients' body fluids, they should wear 2 pairs of disposable gloves (these can be bought at most pharmacies or supermarkets). Even if they wear gloves, they should wash their hands frequently with soap or hand sanitizer.

(3) If a caregiver comes into contact with the patients' body fluids, they should wash the area well with warm water and soap. This will probably not cause any harm, but try to avoid it.

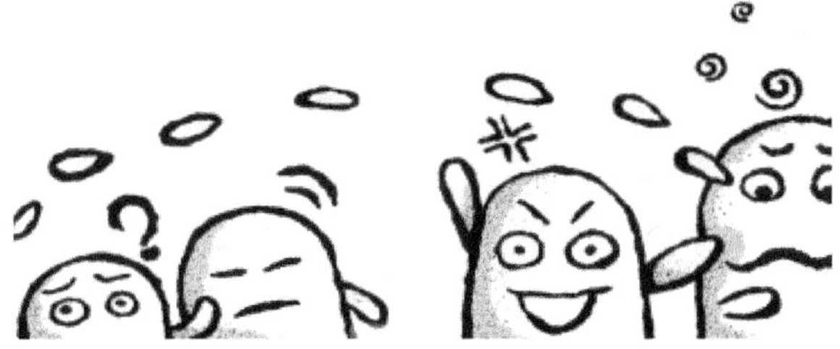

(4) Frequent exposure to crowded places may cause problems and special care should be taken to avoid such exposure.

(5) Wash any clothing or bed linens that have body fluids on them separately and not with other clothes. If you cannot wash these clothes right away, seal them in a plastic bag.

(6) When using disposable adult diapers, underwear or sanitary pads, seal them in two layers of plastic bags and throw them away with regular garbage.

Part 3: What Are the Common Problems in Chemotherapy?

1. What is the difference between radiotherapy and chemotherapy? Patients should choose which one?

Differences between chemotherapy and radiotherapy:

(1) The treatment methods are different: radiotherapy is radiation therapy; chemotherapy is drug therapy.

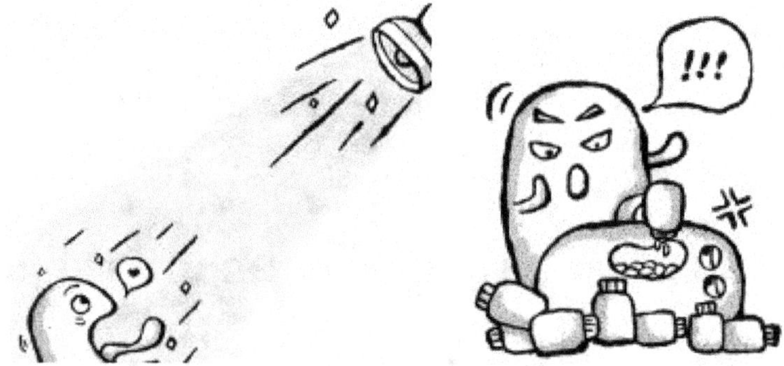

(2) Different side effects: Radiotherapy mostly causes local reactions; chemotherapy causes systemic reactions, which are more severe and more difficult to tolerate than radiotherapy.

(3) Different types of tumors are suitable: Radiotherapy is generally used for tumors in the head and neck, breast, thyroid, and throat. It is not effective for tumors in other parts of the body, while chemotherapy is the opposite.

The above explains the differences between radiotherapy and chemotherapy. Numerous studies have shown that while these two treatments differ, neither is inherently superior to the other. The condition of each patient is different, so the treatment methods adopted are also different. It is impossible to conclude whether radiotherapy or chemotherapy is better. Then, performing radiotherapy and chemotherapy on the same patient is also limited by patients' tumor type and case stage, so it is still impossible to determine whether chemotherapy is better or radiotherapy. In short, patients should follow their doctor's advice and select the most suitable treatment approach.

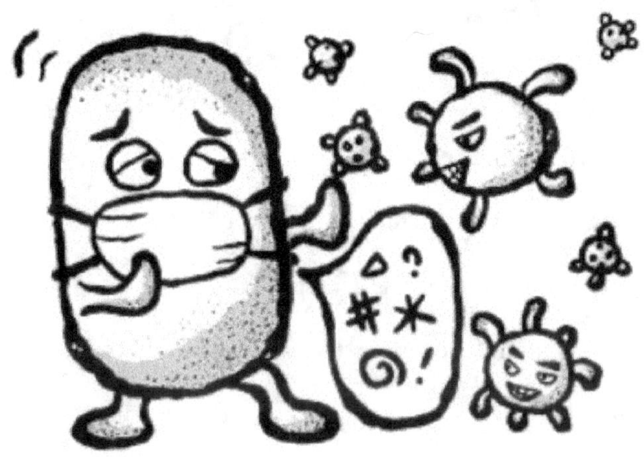

2. What are the main toxic and side effects of chemotherapy drugs?

(1) Nausea and vomiting: These are the most common toxic reactions to chemotherapy drugs, but the severity varies. Chemotherapy drugs that cause severe vomiting include cisplatin (DDP), nitrogen mustard (HN2), doxorubicin (ADM), and epirubicin (EPI), while miltiorrhiza (MMC), bleomycin (BLM), paclitaxel (PTX), and taxotere (TXT) are less likely to

cause nausea and vomiting.

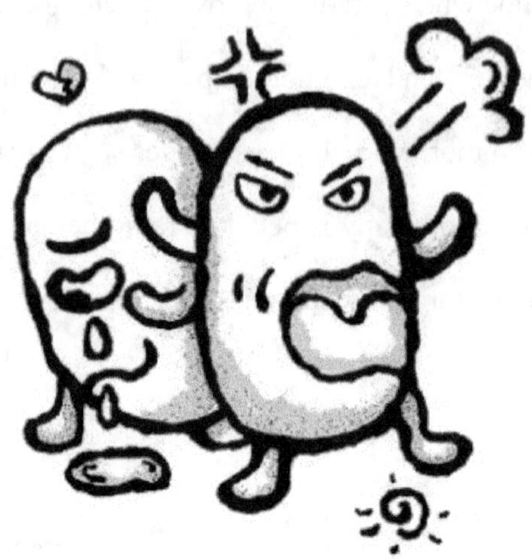

(2) Bone marrow suppression: Most chemotherapy drugs have bone marrow suppression, among which paclitaxel (PTX), taxotere (TXT), vinorelbine (NVB), etoposide (VP-16), carboplatin (CBP), ifosfamide (IFO), methotrexate (MTX), and doxorubicin (ADM) are more obvious. Generally, neutrophil leukopenia occurs first, followed by thrombocytopenia. Mitomycin (MMC) and gemcitabine (GEM) may cause thrombocytopenia first.

(3) Diarrhea: Oxaliplatin (L-OHP), irinotecan (CPT-11), fluorouracil (5-FU), and capecitabine (CAP) may cause diarrhea.

(4) Constipation: Vinorelbine (NVB), vincristine (VCR), vindesine (VDS) and centrally acting antiemetics can all cause constipation.

(5) Cardiotoxicity: Doxorubicin (ADM), epirubicin (EPI), pyrarubicin (THP), and paclitaxel (PTX) are cardiotoxic, which can manifest clinically as chest tightness, weakness, and arrhythmia.

(6) Hair loss: Almost all chemotherapy drugs can cause hair loss, but the severity varies. Mild cases only cause a small amount of hair loss, while

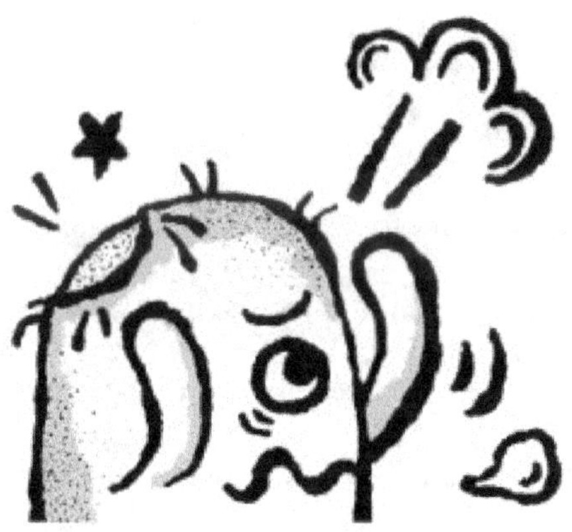

severe cases can cause all hair loss. Doxorubicin (ADM), epirubicin (EPI), pyrarubicin (THP), and paclitaxel (PTX) 100% cause complete hair loss.

(7) Pigmentation: Fluorouracil (5-FU), bleomycin (BLM), and bleomycin (PYM) can cause pigment deposition in the skin and nail beds, resulting in darkening of the skin or nails.

(8) Neurotoxicity: Oxaliplatin (L-OHP), vinorelbine (NVB), paclitaxel (PTX), vincristine (VCR), and etoposide (VP-16) can all produce peripheral neurotoxicity. Patients may experience numbness in the extremities, muscle aches in the limbs, and tingling or numbness in the lips and tongue. In rare

cases, some individuals may develop throat tightness and breathing difficulties, which require immediate medical attention.

(9) Damage to liver and kidney function: Almost all chemotherapy drugs are metabolized by the liver and excreted by the kidneys, so they may damage liver and kidney function. There are also some rare toxic side effects, such as allergies, rashes, and central nervous system toxicity.

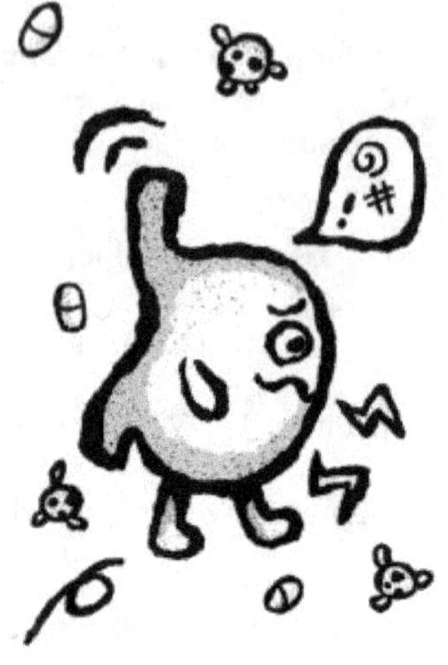

3. Why is chemotherapy still necessary after the malignant tumor has been completely removed surgically?

In clinical practice, most malignant tumors are found to have undergone microscopic metastasis at the time of initial diagnosis. These micrometastases are undetectable by current imaging techniques such as CT, MRI, or B-ultrasound and are referred to as subclinical metastases. It is precisely because of these subclinical metastases that some patients experience tumor recurrence or metastasis some time after surgery.

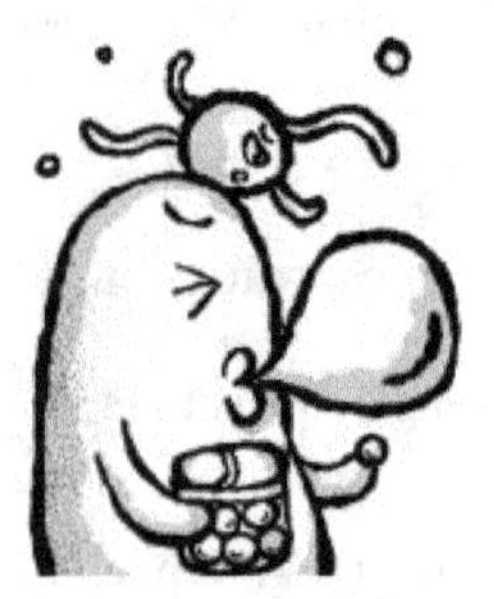

If postoperative follow-up examinations or adjuvant chemotherapy are not performed, the risk of recurrence and metastasis remains high. The danger of malignant tumor cells lies in their resilience—even a few remaining cells can proliferate into widespread metastatic lesions, akin to a single spark starting a prairie fire.

Clinical evidence demonstrates that postoperative adjuvant chemotherapy improves survival rates in most malignant tumors, particularly in patients with intermediate to advanced-stage cancer. The later the tumor is detected, the higher the likelihood of metastasis. Therefore, for patients with advanced-stage malignancies, doctors typically recommend prompt systemic chemotherapy after surgery to eliminate or control these potential micrometastases.

4. Are chemotherapy drugs poisonous?

Chemotherapy drugs, medically termed "cytotoxic agents," are inherently toxic to cells. The hallmark of cancer is uncontrolled cellular proliferation, and these drugs specifically target rapidly dividing cells, inducing their death. Thus, referring to chemotherapy drugs as "poisons" is not an exaggeration.

Although cytotoxic agents are highly toxic, cancer cells typically divide faster than normal cells, making them more susceptible to the drugs' effects. However, chemotherapy lacks selectivity—it cannot distinguish between malignant and healthy cells. Consequently, normal cells with high proliferation rates (such as bone marrow cells and hair follicle cells) are also affected, leading to common side effects like myelosuppression and hair loss.

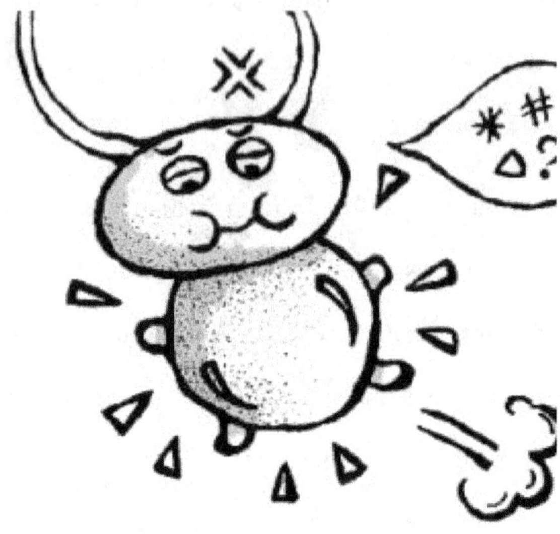

5. Is it correct to say that since chemotherapy drugs are poisons and may hasten patients' death, it is better not to take them?

There are strict criteria for determining whether a patient is suitable for chemotherapy. Even if a patient requests it, chemotherapy will not be administered if their overall health is compromised. This is because chemotherapy carries significant side effects, and if the patient cannot tolerate them, proceeding with treatment would only worsen their condition and cause additional harm.

Some claim that chemotherapy increases cancer mortality rates, but this is an oversimplification. Treatment suitability depends entirely on the patient's specific condition. For example, a colorectal cancer patient with intestinal obstruction, inability to eat, and severely compromised health would undoubtedly deteriorate further with chemotherapy. In such cases, chemotherapy offers no benefit and only imposes unnecessary risks.

Thus, the key lies in selecting the right patients for the right treatment.

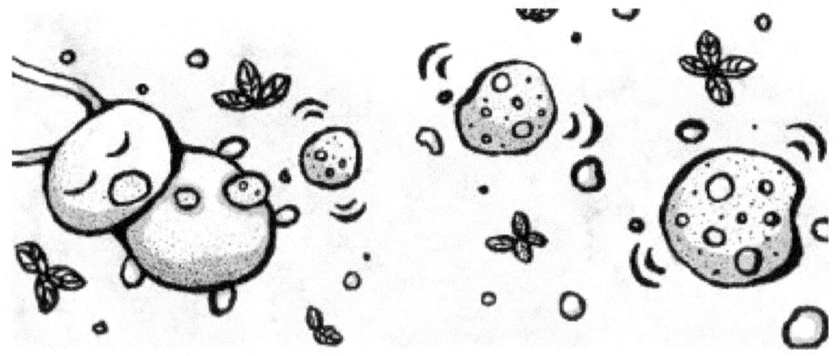

6. Does chemotherapy have to kill all cancer cells?

In cancer treatment, public perception often polarizes into two extremes. One view claims that cancer is incurable—arguing that even with treatment, patients will die sooner—so they suggest "eat well and wait for death at home." The other extreme insists that cancer must be eradicated at all costs, pushing chemotherapy to its limits with the mentality of "as long as there's life, there's chemotherapy

Both views are misguided. While chemotherapy is indeed essential for advanced cancer, it is not a limitless battle. The goal should be to strike a balance—maximizing therapeutic efficacy while minimizing toxic side effects. Thus, chemotherapy must be personalized—administered judiciously, tailored to the patient's condition, and stopped when risks outweigh benefits.

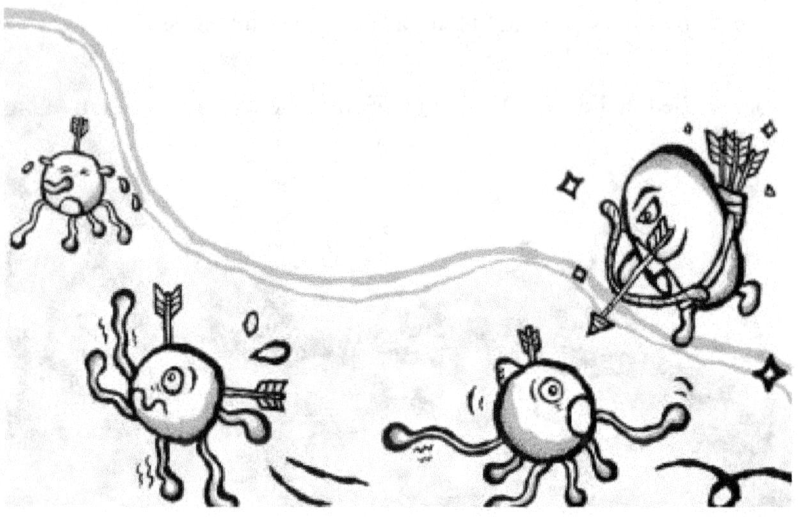

7. Are all elderly people unable to tolerate chemotherapy?

Cancer is more common among the elderly, and many of them do not undergo chemotherapy due to their age, which results in many elderly patients who need chemotherapy losing the opportunity to receive chemotherapy. In fact, whether or not one can tolerate chemotherapy depends not only on age, but also on a person's biological age. Many elderly patients can tolerate chemotherapy because of their good physical condition.

8. Do all patients with malignant tumors need chemotherapy?

The answer is no. Whether a malignant tumor patient requires chemotherapy requires a comprehensive analysis. Chemotherapy is divided into: neoadjuvant chemotherapy, adjuvant chemotherapy, and palliative chemotherapy. Many patients with early malignant tumors do not need chemotherapy.

9. Why do chemotherapy patients need to have their blood checked regularly?

After chemotherapy, blood tests are required every 2 to 3 days. Some patients do not understand this and think: "My blood results were normal last time - why repeat the test?" In fact, regular blood tests are very necessary. Many current chemotherapy regimens may cause bone marrow suppression, which is mainly manifested by a decrease in white blood cells (mainly neutrophils) and some also have a decrease in platelets. Generally, white blood cells tend to decrease from the first day of chemotherapy and remain in a suppressed state until the 14th day (some regimens even until the 20th day). Bone marrow suppression is graded as:

Grade I: $3.0\text{-}4.0\times10^9/L$

Grade II: $2.0\text{-}3.0\times10^9/L$

Grade III: $1.0\text{-}2.0\times10^9/L$

Grade IV: $<1.0\times10^9/L$

Patients with grade III and IV bone marrow suppression are at risk of causing severe infection and leading to death. Platelets $< 30\times10^9/L$ are at risk of spontaneous bleeding. Everyone has a different tolerance to chemotherapy, and the time, degree and duration of bone marrow suppression are also different. Some appear on the 2nd or 3rd day of chemotherapy, while others appear on the 10th day; some are only grade I, while others may have 0 white blood cells; some are normal the day before, and become grade III the next day. Therefore, according to the chemotherapy regimen, patients' age, physical condition, and previous chemotherapy, it is necessary for patients to have a routine blood test every 2 to 3 days.

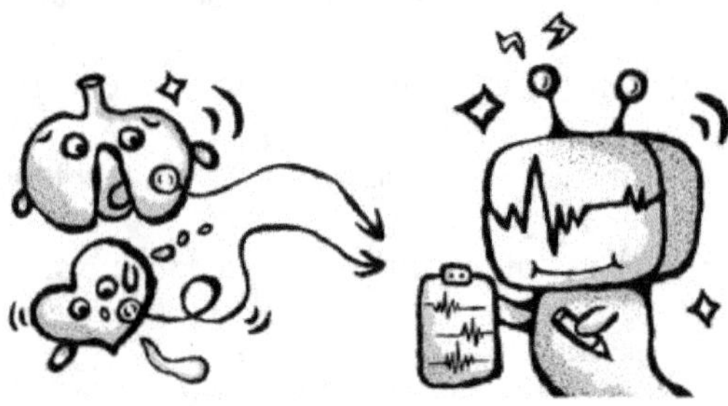

10. What to do when white blood cell count drops after chemotherapy?

Chemotherapy drugs can cause varying degrees of leukocytopenia. Patients should avoid wind chill, be careful about their daily life, reduce going out and visiting, and try to avoid colds. Because the cellular immune function is low at this time, colds may be complicated by difficult-to-control bacterial infections. Leukocytopenia above degree II should be promptly treated with recombinant human granulocyte colony-stimulating factor to promote bone marrow function recovery and reduce the chance of severe infection. Blood routine tests should be performed every day or every other day during the use of recombinant human granulocyte colony-stimulating

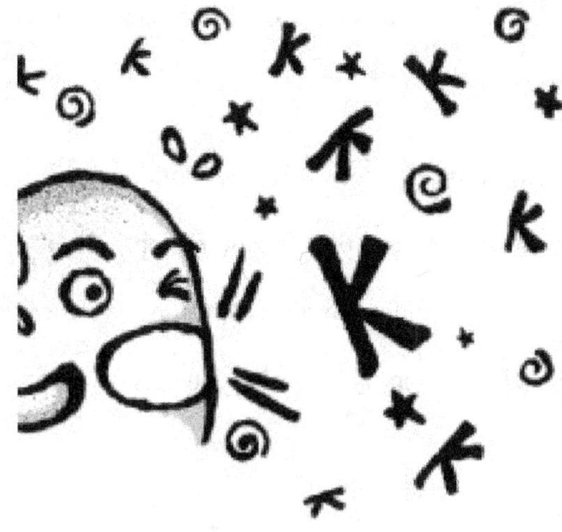

factor. Some patients' white blood cells rose rapidly to more than 10×10^9/L on the second and third days of using recombinant human granulocyte colony-stimulating factor. This is because the granulocytes stored in the peripheral bone marrow pool are released into the blood. The real bone marrow hematopoietic function has not yet recovered. It is necessary to continue using it until the blood routine white blood cell count is more than 10×10^9/L again. The chance of infection with grade IV bone marrow suppression is very high. At this time, patients should do a good job of self-isolation, reduce visiting, ensure personal hygiene and food hygiene, ensure air circulation in the ward, cooperate with nurses to measure body temperature on time, and notify doctors and nurses in time if fever, oral ulcers, sore throat, diarrhea, etc. are found. But there is no need to worry too much. Generally, with the help of recombinant human granulocyte colony-stimulating factor, most patients can return to normal within a week.

11. What to do when suffering nausea and vomiting during chemotherapy?

Most chemotherapy drugs cause varying degrees of nausea and vomiting. Agents like cisplatin, carboplatin, doxorubicin, and epirubicin are particularly emetogenic (likely to induce nausea and vomiting), which is a major reason many patients fear chemotherapy. So, how can this discomfort be alleviated?

First, patients still have to trust doctors. Oncologists who have undergone good professional training will standardize the use of antiemetics when using drugs that cause patients to vomit at medium/intensity. Some also add glucocorticoids and sedatives, which can greatly reduce the degree of nausea and vomiting. Patients should relax their bodies and minds. They can listen to music, watch TV or books, and chat with others during chemotherapy to avoid focusing too much on chemotherapy. Individuals have different degrees of reaction to chemotherapy drugs, so some people still have nausea and vomiting under strong antiemetic treatment. If vomiting occurs more than 3 times, doctors and nurses should be notified in time and give treatment such as metoclopramide. During chemotherapy, do not pursue nutrition in the diet. Take "want to eat and be able to eat" as the standard. The food should be as light as possible and easy to digest. Semi-liquid food is better, and small meals are eaten frequently. Patients can eat porridge and egg custard. These semi-liquid foods can form a protective film on the surface of the esophagus and stomach, reducing the damage of gastric juice to the upper digestive tract.

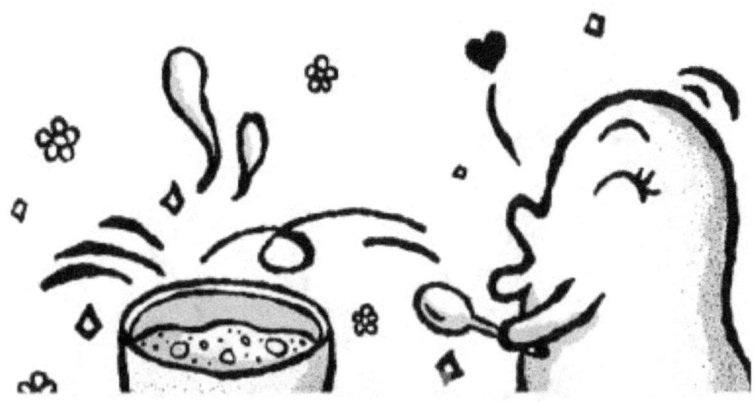

12. What to do when suffering from constipation during chemotherapy?

Constipation is prone to occur during chemotherapy. First, chemotherapy drugs such as vinorelbine, vincristine, and vindesine have the side effect of constipation; second, the large-scale use of central antiemetic drugs will inhibit intestinal peristalsis and cause constipation; third, exercise and diet are reduced during chemotherapy, and the intake of fewer vegetables and fruits can also easily lead to constipation. Constipation prevention is more important than treatment. When using chemotherapy drugs that cause constipation, Traditional Chinese Medicine that moisturizes the intestines and promotes bowel movements can be taken, such as Ma Ren Runchang Pills and Compound Aloe Capsules, and eat some fruits and vegetables that have a laxative effect, such as bananas, kiwis, spinach, etc. Patients who can get out of bed should try to get out of bed and walk around. Patients with poor physical strength can massage their abdomen from left to right in bed to promote intestinal peristalsis. Acupuncture and moxibustion also have good results in treating constipation.

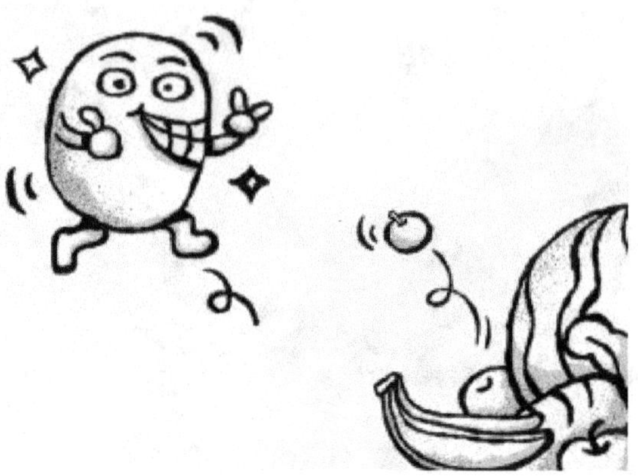

13. What to do when suffering diarrhea during chemotherapy?

Chemotherapy drugs such as fluorouracil, oxaliplatin, irinotecan, and capecitabine may accelerate intestinal peristalsis and increase secretions, leading to chemotherapy-induced diarrhea. Addition-ally, damage to the intestinal mucosa by these drugs, combined with an unhygienic diet, can trigger infectious diarrhea. Therefore, patients during chemotherapy should pay attention to bowel

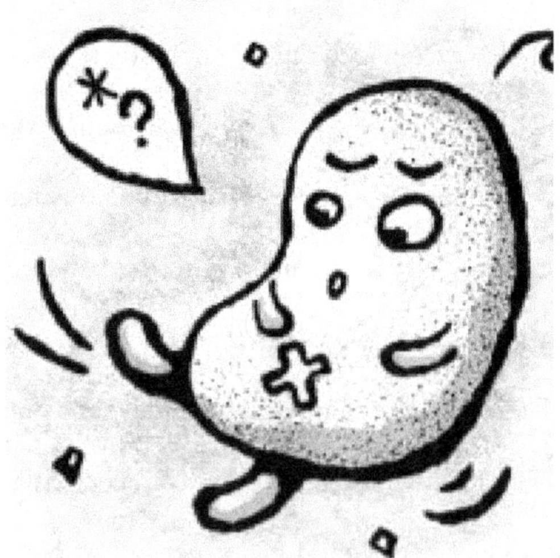

movement. If the number of bowel movements increases an/or the stool becomes thinner, do not take medicine in private, and inform doctors in time. First of all, it is necessary to distinguish between infectious diarrhea and chemotherapy diarrhea, and routine stool examination is essential. Antidiarrheal drugs such as Imodium can be used for chemotherapy diarrhea, but antidiarrheal drugs cannot be used for infectious diarrhea, and antibiotics should be used immediately. Patients should drink plenty of water to replenish water and electrolytes, and intravenous fluid and potassium supplements when necessary; the diet must be light and non-greasy, mainly carbohydrates, and try to drink less gas-producing foods such as milk and soy milk; the anus and vulva should be cleaned in time after defecation to prevent bacterial infection.

14. How to reduce the neurotoxic response to chemotherapy?

Oxaliplatin, vinorelbine, paclitaxel, docetaxel, vinca alkaloids, etoposide, etc., can all produce peripheral neurotoxicity, which is mainly manifested as numbness of hands and feet, and muscle soreness in the limbs. It can 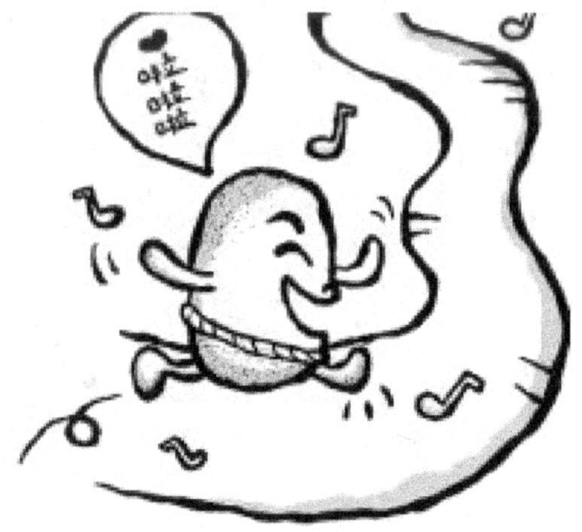 occur during chemotherapy, or it can gradually appear and worsen as the chemotherapy course increases. How to reduce neurotoxicity? The most important thing is to avoid cold drinks and cold food during chemotherapy, and also avoid contact between hands and feet and cold objects. It is best to wear cotton socks and thin gloves when using oxaliplatin. Supplementing B vitamins during chemotherapy can nourish the nerves and reduce drug damage to the nerves. Chinese medicine for external use to soak hands and feet can promote local blood circulation, increase nerve nutrition, and accelerate the repair of nerve damage.

15. How long after chemotherapy can patients take a shower?

Patients can safely bathe during chemotherapy. Bathing can remove dirt from the skin, make people more comfortable, and reduce the adverse reactions of radiotherapy and chemotherapy. At the same time, bathing will not reduce the effects of radiotherapy and chemotherapy. It is very important to pay attention to the water temperature and timely warming measures, because chemotherapy will cause a weak constitution and poor immunity, and it is easier to catch colds and other diseases. While such illnesses are typically mild

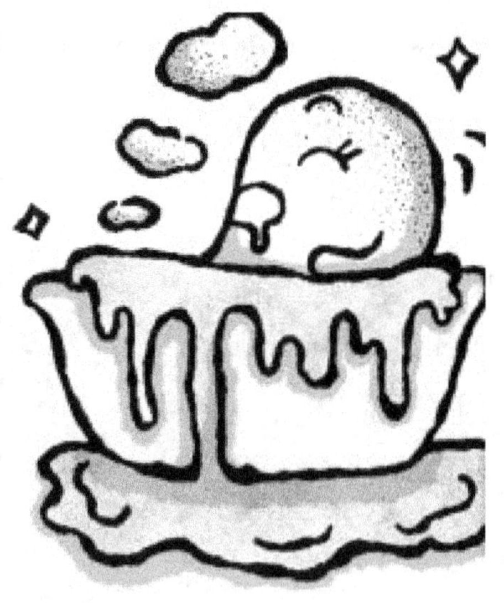

for healthy individuals, they pose significant risks to chemotherapy patients.

16. Will chemotherapy definitely cause nausea and vomiting?

Most people think that chemotherapy is definitely accompanied by gastrointestinal reactions such as nausea and vomiting, but this is not the case. Although nausea and vomiting are among the most common adverse reactions of chemotherapy drugs, there are many factors that cause nausea and vomiting clinically, which can involve diseases and lesions of multiple systems in the body. Moreover, the emetic effects and emetic mechanisms of various chemotherapy drugs, as well as the time and duration of vomiting after medication are not the same. According to the probability of vomiting reactions caused by anti-tumor drugs, the risks of vomiting reactions caused by various drugs are divided into four levels. Specific classification: high-level: cisplatin, nitrogen mustard, cyclophosphamide, etc.; intermediate: oxaliplatin, carboplatin, cytarabine, etc.; low-level: paclitaxel, docetaxel, etc.; very low-level: vinorelbine, bleomycin, etc. So not all chemotherapy drugs will cause nausea and vomiting.

17. Do chemotherapy drugs cause hair loss? What to do if so?

Certain chemotherapy drugs may cause alopecia (hair loss). While chemotherapy-induced hair loss poses no direct health risks, it can significantly impact patients' appearance and self-image. To help manage this side effect, we recommend that patients: Cut their hair short before starting chemotherapy; reduce the number of times they comb their hair, and delay the time of hair loss.

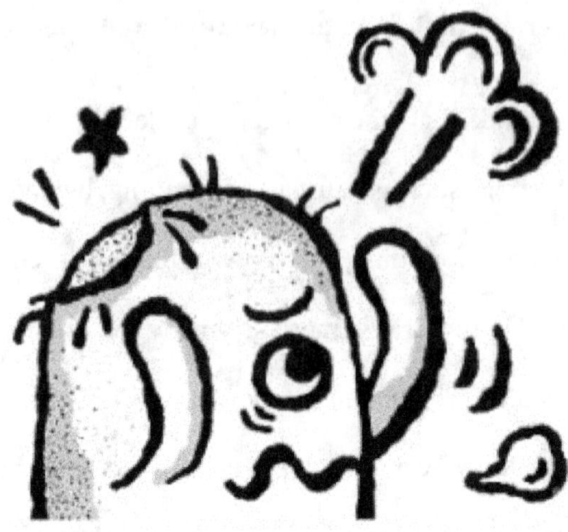

18. What to do when experiencing numbness in fingers and toes after chemotherapy?

Chemotherapy patients may experience numbness and paresthesia in their fingers and toes after using chemotherapy drugs. For example, "paclitaxel" can cause paresthesia in peripheral nerves, which mainly affects pain and temperature sensation.

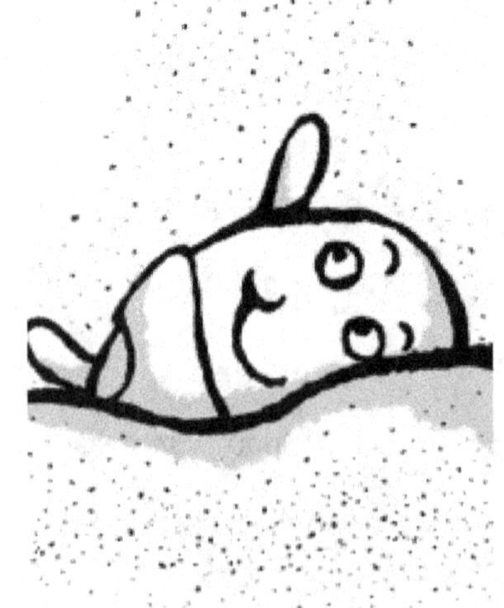

When this symptom occurs, drugs can be used to nourish nerves, soak the hands and feet in warm water to relieve the numbness, and do appropriate hand and foot massage and acupuncture treatment to speed up the recovery process.

In daily life, attention should be paid

to avoid touching overheated objects. For example, when holding a hot water cup, we can keep our fingernails and touch it first to avoid burns and other adverse events due to slow reaction of fingers touching objects. Avoid contact with sharp objects, such as doing needlework (cross stitch) to avoid punctures.

19. Can family and friends be around during chemotherapy?

Most chemotherapy drugs can lower patients' resistance to infection, so they should take steps to avoid infection. Stay away from anyone who is sick. It is necessary for them to wash their hands often, especially before touching their face, nose, mouth, or eyes. When they are with their family, family and friends need to do the same.

Rarely will chemotherapy require patients to avoid close contact with loved ones for a short period of time, but if necessary, talk to doctors when making treatment choices. Make sure patients stay up to date on their vaccinations. Flu shots are especially important because people with cancer are at high risk for serious flu complications. Talk to doctors about which vaccine is right for patients. Infections can 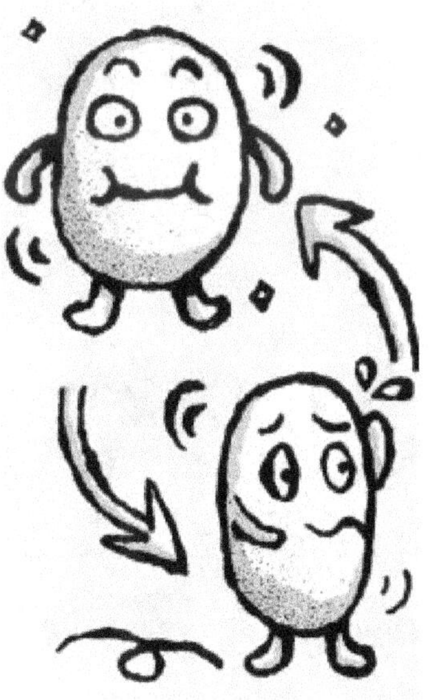 also occur from food and drinks, so food safety is very important when the immune system is weak. Talk to doctors about whether patients need to follow a special diet during cancer treatment. Some pets can also spread infections, so be sure to keep them healthy and take precautions when they are around.

20. What to do when catching a cold during chemotherapy?

Patients must first distinguish the type of cold. In Traditional Chinese Medicine, there are two types of colds: wind-cold colds and wind-heat colds. Without distinguishing them, taking medicine for wind-heat colds or taking medicine for wind-cold colds will not effectively treat the cold. Moreover, if the bacterial or viral infection is severe, intravenous anti-infection treatment is required.

In the early stage of a cold, patients can drink plenty of water and get adequate rest to boost their immunity. Medication can be taken on the third day if necessary. Eat light food, such as porridge, noodle soup, fresh vegetables and fruits. Avoid eating greasy, cold, sour and fishy foods (such as rice dumplings, ice cream, chocolate, stale seafood, etc.). Keep warm and avoid rain or water to avoid catching a cold again.

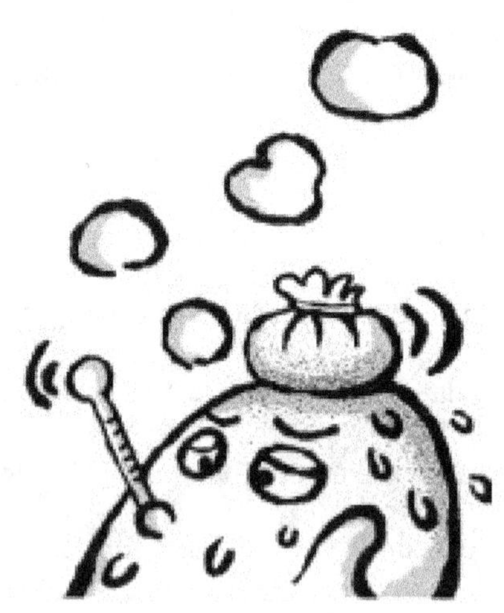

After recovering from a cold, patients can choose the following foods:

(1) High-protein diet: It mainly improves the body's resistance and provides a material basis for the recovery of white blood cells to normal. High-protein foods include poultry eggs, lean meat, animal liver, kidney, milk, beans and their products.

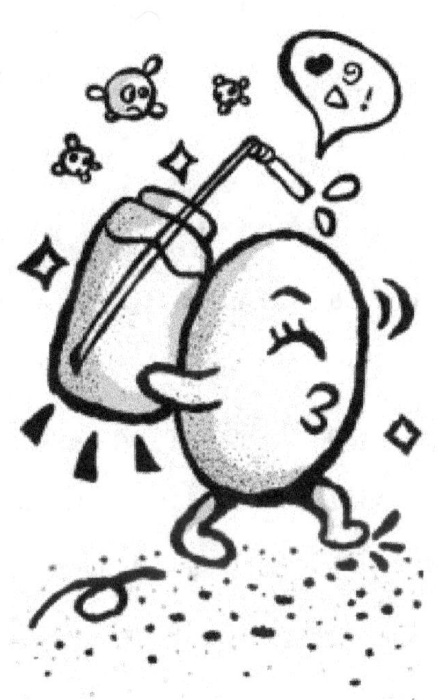

(2) High-vitamin diet: Vitamins can promote cell growth and development. They help differentiate and proliferate white blood cells and promote recovery to normal. High-vitamin foods should include yeast-raised foods, cereals, peanuts, fresh green fruits, fruit juices, etc., to supplement vitamin C, B vitamins, and folic acid. Since patients are prone to infections, all foods should be strictly disinfected during preparation, and raw, cold, or unclean foods should be avoided.

21. What happens if the fever doesn't go away after chemotherapy?

Chemotherapy suppresses white blood cell production, reducing the number of these infection-fighting cells and significantly increasing the risk of infection. This condition often leads to infectious complications. Chemotherapy itself has significant side effects, commonly causing nausea, vomiting, hair loss, loss of appetite, leukopenia (low white blood cell count), and weakened immunity. While destroying cancer cells, it also damages a large number of healthy cells and may, to some extent, even promote cancer cell growth. Fever after chemotherapy may occur due to the patient's weakened immune state. Viruses, bacteria, or their metabolites stimulate the release of endogenous substances like prostaglandins. These substances act on the body's thermoregulatory center, raising its set point and resulting in elevated body temperature.

The main reasons why patients have persistent fever after chemotherapy are: on the one hand, cancer cells affect the body's ability to regulate body temperature; on the other hand, most patients will have decreased immunity due to the tumor itself or treatment, especially patients with low white blood cells, who often have fever due to infection. In addition, drug reactions, autoimmune diseases, insufficient secretion of adrenal cortex hormones or cancer itself can cause fever. In such cases, physical cooling can only provide temporary relief. Traditional Chinese Medicine is recommended for syndrome differentiation and holistic treatment. Traditional Chinese Medicine has the functions of clearing away heat and detoxifying, strengthening the body and eliminating evil, improving the body's immunity, and improving patients' fever symptoms.

22. Will everything be fine after chemotherapy?

The current medical consensus is that endless chemotherapy is harmful and useless, so chemotherapy generally has a limited course of treatment. The most commonly used clinical regimen is a 21- to 28-day cycle. Postoperative adjuvant chemotherapy is generally performed for 4 to 6 cycles, and advanced patients are generally 3 to 6 cycles. The 14-day regimen is generally performed for 10 to 12 cycles. Some patients breathe a sigh of relief after the end of conventional chemotherapy: "Finally, it's over." Is it "cured" after the end of the chemotherapy course? No. The development of malignant tumors is a long and gradual process, and the treatment of malignant tumors is also long-term. Chemotherapy is only one step in the treatment. After chemotherapy, Chinese herbal decoctions or finished medicines can be taken for a long time, which can help to support the body's vitality and detoxify and disperse the knots. After chemotherapy, a comprehensive review should be conducted every 3 to 6 months to detect recurrence and metastasis in time.

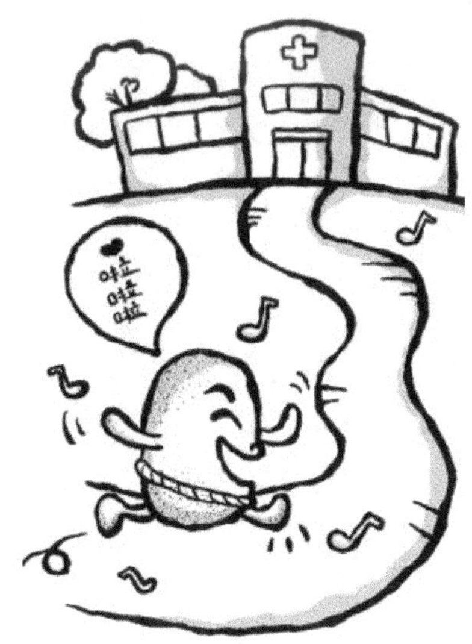

Part 4: What to Eat During Chemotherapy?

During the whole chemotherapy process, if there is no reasonable and sufficient nutrition guarantee, the treatment plan will not be implemented smoothly. Therefore, whether in the hospital or at home, dietary care cannot be ignored. The dietary principles for cancer

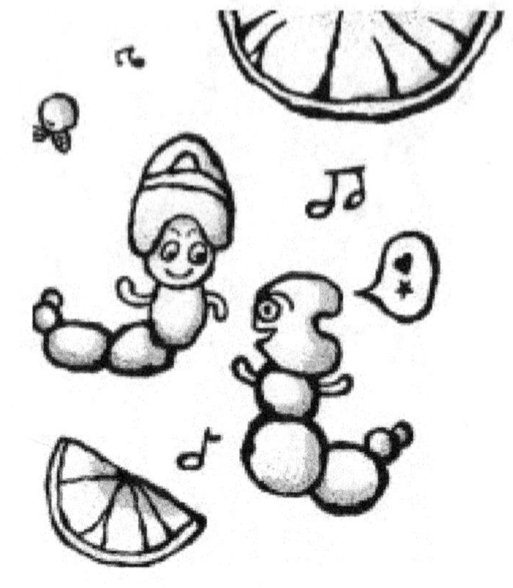

patients emphasize a light, high-calorie, high-vitamin, and low-fat diet. Enhancing food flavors with sweet and sour seasonings can help stimulate appetite while alleviating chemotherapy-induced nausea, vomiting, and loss of appetite.

1. Dietary principles for patients in chemotherapy

Food should be diversified as much as possible. Eat more high-protein, vitamin-rich, low-animal fat, and easily digestible foods, along with fresh fruits and vegetables. Do not eat stale, spoiled or irritating foods, do not eat carbonated drinks and other gas-producing foods, eat less smoked, grilled, pickled, fried, and overly salty foods, and combine coarse and fine grains in staple foods to ensure nutritional balance and prevent bloating, diarrhea and constipation.

To prevent the decrease of white blood cells and platelets caused by chemotherapy, it is advisable to eat more blood and meat, such as animal offal, egg yolks, lean meat, fish, eel, chicken, bones, etc.; at the same time, patients can also take medicated food, such as Codonopsis pilosula, Astragalus membranaceus, Angelica sinensis, red dates, peanuts, etc.

To improve immune function, patients can eat foods such as shiitake mushrooms, mushrooms, Hericium erinaceus, and black fungus.

To stimulate appetite and reduce nausea/vomiting, patients can try the following dietary adjustments: Modify meal composition and cooking methods to enhance food's color, aroma, and flavor; eat small meals frequently, and eat some light and refreshing raw cold dishes; add some ginger to the diet to stop vomiting; patients can also use medicated food to stimulate the appetite and strengthen the spleen, such as diced hawthorn and meat, astragalus, yam, radish, tangerine peel, etc.

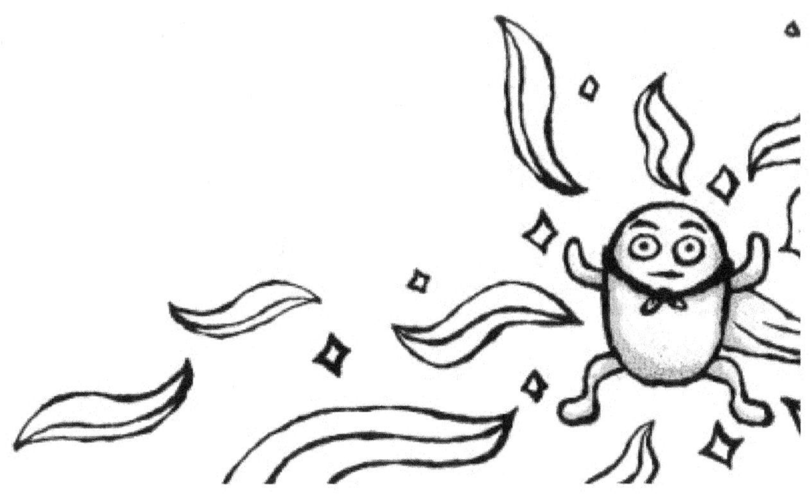

2. Diet during chemotherapy

1. Chemotherapy interval

Patients should eat a high-protein, high-vitamin diet, such as lean meat, beef, boneless fish, boneless ribs, etc. They should also eat more fresh vegetables and fruits. Pay attention to food hygiene, wash fruits and vegetables, eat fresh food, and do not eat spoiled food.

2. During chemotherapy

(1) The diet should be light, low in residue, easily digestible and less irritating. Greasy, rough and prickly foods should be avoided to avoid damaging the oral and gastrointestinal mucosa.

(2) If patients feel nauseous during chemotherapy, they can eat a small amount, but they must not stop eating.

(3) Eat small meals frequently. If patients are taking oral chemotherapy drugs, there should be a gap between meal times and medication times, with a minimum interval of 2 hours.

(4) Between meals, patients can eat some foods that are not likely to cause nausea, such as crackers, biscuits, fresh fruits, etc. Chew them slowly to avoid injuring the oral mucosa.

(5) Take good care of oral cavity before and after meals.

(6) If feeling severe nausea, patients should reduce activities and stop

eating. Deep breaths can be taken repeatedly to relieve the discomfort.

(7) Family members often provide patients with their favorite food.

(8) When oral ulcers occur, the diet should mainly consist of semi-liquid or liquid foods, such as milk, vegetable porridge, soy milk, noodles, etc.

(9) Eat more fresh fruits, and peel them. Fruits and raw vegetables that cannot be eaten include peaches, bananas, grapes, cucumbers, tomatoes, lychees, plums, and strawberries. Some of these fruits have hairs and are difficult to clean; some have rough skins and are difficult to disinfect; and some have thin skins that are easily damaged, making it easy for bacteria to invade and multiply. Fruits that can be eaten should have skins that are not damaged or rotten, such as watermelons, apples, pears, tangerines, and oranges.

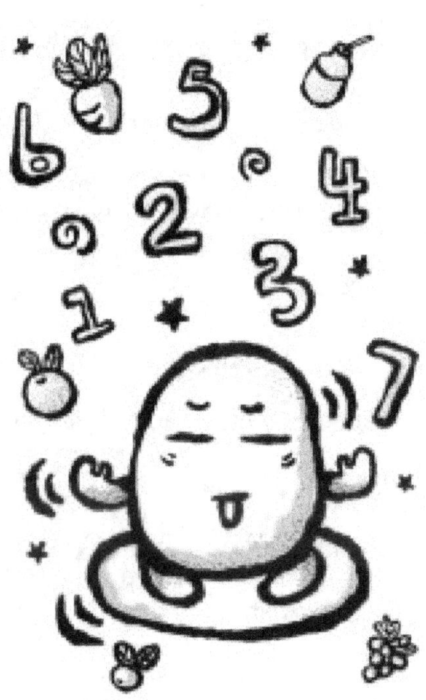

(10) During chemotherapy, drink plenty of water and non-irritating liquids, such as fruit juice, to promote the excretion of metabolic products in the body and reduce side effects.

3. Early end of chemotherapy

Patients should gradually increase food intake, focusing on high-protein and vitamin-rich foods like chicken, beef, lamb, and celery. However, avoid hard-to-digest foods (e.g., roast duck) to prevent diarrhea. Incorporate plenty of fresh fruits and vegetables, and maintain strict food hygiene to reduce the risk of gastrointestinal infections.

3. Suggestions for three-meal-a-day dietary for chemotherapy patients

1. Breakfast: light and easy to digest

The saying 'eat a good breakfast' holds particular importance for chemotherapy patients. While maintaining good nutrition, their diet should be carefully tailored to their condition. Given their weakened digestive function, an ideal breakfast might include easily digestible steamed egg custard, paired 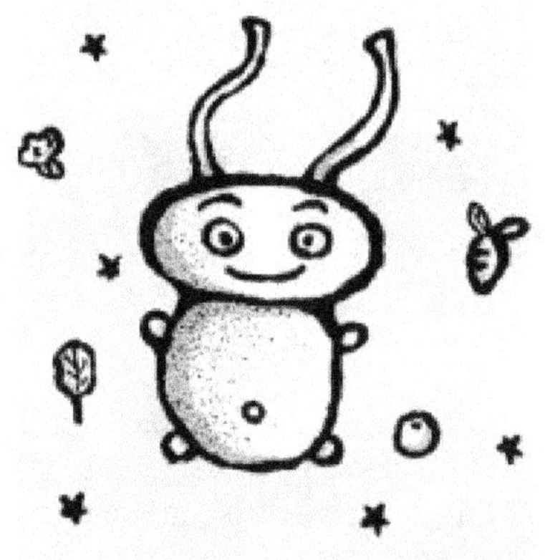 with a small steamed bun or cake, a bowl of whole grain porridge, and a glass of milk - providing both optimal nutrition and gentle digestion.

2. Lunch: A combination of meat and vegetables, mainly nutritious

As the saying goes, "Eat a hearty meal at noon." For healthy individuals, daily nutritional needs should be replenished promptly. However, for chemotherapy patients, simply replenishing calories isn't enough—careful dietary choices are essential. A balanced combination of meat and vegetables, along with nutrient-rich foods, is most important. For patients with poor digestion, a bowl of noodles can be a good option. Consider adding minced meat (finely chopped for easier digestion), along with some chopped vegetables. Additionally, 100g of fish and a few side dishes can provide a well-rounded, easily digestible meal.

3. Dinner: light and nutritious

As the saying goes, "Eat light at night"—and this applies to chemotherapy patients as well. However, patients need to ensure the intake of nutrients on this basis. Both chemotherapy and the disease itself consume energy. It is difficult to eat less and ensure the intake of nutrients when patients cannot eat for a long time at night. For dinner, a light but nourishing option is minced meat porridge: simply add finely minced meat to plain rice porridge. A serving of 100–150 grams of porridge, paired with a glass of milk and some vegetables (such as fish, meat, or leafy greens), can provide balanced nutrition without overburdening digestion.

4. Five fruits suitable for eating after chemotherapy

1. Grapes

Resveratrol contained in grapes can prevent normal cells from becoming cancerous and inhibit the spread of already malignant cells. Chinese medicine believes that grapes can replenish Qi and blood, relieve restlessness and thirst, and strengthen the stomach and promote urination. Sweet and sour grapes are more suitable for cancer patients who have undergone radiotherapy or surgery and can be eaten regularly.

2. Blackcurrant

Blackcurrant is a wild fruit that grows in the northeast of my country. It has high nutritional and health value. Its fruit is rich in vitamin C and its protein content ranks first among the wild fruits known in China. In particular, its juice can block the synthesis of carcinogen nitrosamine morpholine. It can block the formation of nitrosamines and play an anti-cancer and cancer prevention role.

3. Kiwi

Kiwi fruit is sour, sweet, cold, non-toxic, and has the functions of clearing heat, diuresis, dispersing blood stasis, promoting blood circulation, promoting lactation, and anti-inflammatory. It is rich in vitamin C. Among all fruits in the world, kiwi fruit has the highest absorption rate of vitamin C, which can reach 94%. Vitamin C has anti-cancer effects.

4. Strawberries

Strawberries contain ellagic acid, which can protect the body from carcinogens and have a certain anti-cancer effect. Strawberries have the function of promoting body fluid and quenching thirst, relieving throat and moistening lungs, and are beneficial for relieving radiotherapy reactions and reducing symptoms in patients with nasopharyngeal cancer, lung cancer, and laryngeal cancer.

5. Figs

Pharmacological studies have shown that its dried fruits, unripe fruits and plant juices all contain anti-tumor components, and the latex contains starch saccharifying enzymes, proteases, etc. The dried fruit water extract has an anti-Ehrlich sarcoma effect after being treated with activated carbon and acetone. The unripe fruit latex can inhibit rat transplanted sarcoma and mouse spontaneous breast cancer, causing tumor necrosis, and can also delay the development and degeneration of transplanted adenocarcinoma, bone marrow leukemia, and lymphosarcoma. This product has a wide range of anti-cancer effects and is non-toxic. It tastes

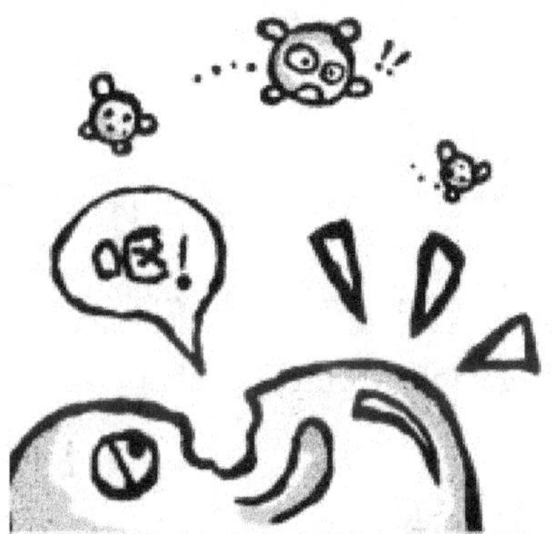

sweet and can be eaten fresh as a fruit. Japan has made injections that are widely used for laryngeal cancer, adenocarcinoma, cervical cancer, bladder cancer, etc.; Traditional Chinese Medicine has also long had records of figs' anti-cancer effects (figs are taken orally in water without restriction, 3 times a day, to treat pyloric cancer; 30 g of figs and 15 g of Akebia are decocted and taken once a day to treat bladder cancer).

It should be noted that the intake of fruit should be controlled and not too much fruit should be consumed in a day, otherwise it will easily cause other types of complications.

5. Diet during different cancer chemotherapy periods

1. Lung cancer patients

Chemotherapy for lung cancer frequently induces gastrointestinal toxicity, adversely affecting treatment compliance and therapeutic outcomes. To mitigate these effects, patients should be encouraged to eat small, frequent meals consisting of light, easily digestible foods. Liquid and semi-liquid foods with low fiber content are recommended, while spicy, cold, hard, and greasy foods should be avoided. Since chemotherapy drugs can cause leukopenia, a diet rich in protein, iron, and vitamins—such as animal liver, lean meat, jujube, longan, donkey-hide gelatin, and fresh fruits and vegetables—is essential. For patients suffering from appetite loss, indigestion, or diarrhea, incorporating spleen- and stomach-nourishing foods like coix seed, white lentils, and jujube can be beneficial.

In cases of severe reactions or prolonged nutritional intake disorders, parenteral nutrition may be necessary to improve the patient's condition. Notably, during the third chemotherapy cycle, appetite loss becomes more pronounced. Relying solely on intravenous supplementation is insufficient to meet energy demands and may hinder recovery. To support digestion and stimulate appetite, oral multi-enzyme tablets can be administered as an adjunct measure.

Encourage patients to eat. For patients with severe vomiting, pay attention to the frequency, amount and color of vomiting, and use antiemetic treatment. For patients with liver damage, they should rest in bed, eat small and frequent meals, and eat nutritious and easily digestible food.

Patients with lung cancer are weak after chemotherapy. It is advisable to choose nutritious and easy-to-digest foods, such as soft rice, porridge, bread, steamed buns, fish, eggs, chicken, soup, potatoes, bananas, jam, etc. The diet should use some light and refreshing foods with little or no oil or some acidic

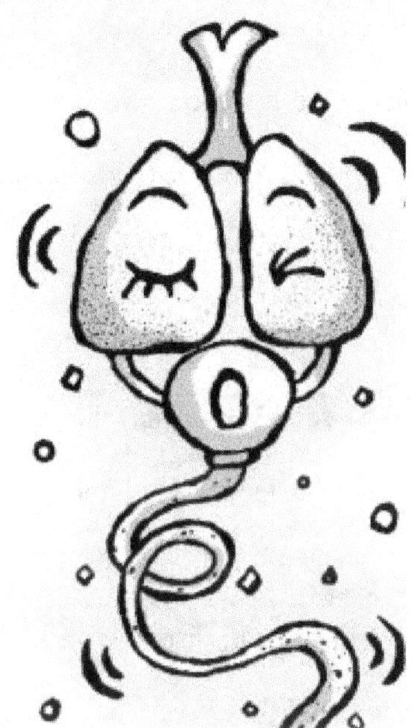

foods, which can stimulate the appetite. Avoid eating spicy, fried, greasy, pickled, and smoked foods. If the weight loss is obvious, then an acidic diet can be used. Use yogurt instead of milk to avoid abdominal bloating and exercise appropriately.

2. Liver cancer patients

Eat more high-calorie, high-protein, high-vitamin and appropriate amounts of inorganic salts and trace elements. Such as rice, noodles, grains, beans, fish, lean meat, eggs, dairy products and soy products, as well as fresh vegetables, fruits, nuts, etc. However, due to liver dysfunction and liver decompensation in patients with liver cancer, such patients should follow doctors' advice and limit the intake of water and salt. When preparing meals, patients' eating habits should be taken into consideration as much as possible. The food temperature should be moderate, and it is not advisable to eat too cold or too hot food. If the toxic side effects during chemotherapy for liver cancer are severe, patients can eat liquid or semi-liquid diets 5 to 6 times a day, such as soy milk, milk, yogurt, egg custard, turtle soup, crucian carp soup, etc.

Diversify patients' diet and pay attention to dietary matching, so that various nutrients complement each other and improve the body's immunity. Prioritize cooking methods like steaming, boiling, or stewing, and emphasize appealing color, aroma, and flavor in meals. Avoid or limit smoked, fried, grilled, and pickled foods. Alcohol and smoking are strictly discouraged, as alcohol may activate carcinogens and weaken immune function. The staple food of liver cancer patients during chemotherapy can be selected according to their eating habits and tastes, such as steamed buns, dumplings, wontons, noodles, etc. Patients with poor appetite can eat small meals more often.

Eat more fresh vegetables and fruits. Studies have found that vegetables are rich in anti-cancer substances, such as cabbage, green onions, garlic, white radish, etc. Patients should eat more foods rich in carotene, vitamin C, and vitamin A, such as celery, cauliflower, leeks, lettuce, garlic sprouts, carrots, onions, tomatoes, etc. In addition, soybeans contain rich nutrients such as fat, protein, minerals, vitamin E, phospholipids and unsaturated fatty acids, so they can eat more of them. Fruits such as watermelon, bananas, oranges, peaches, pineapples, hawthorns, strawberries, kiwis, etc.

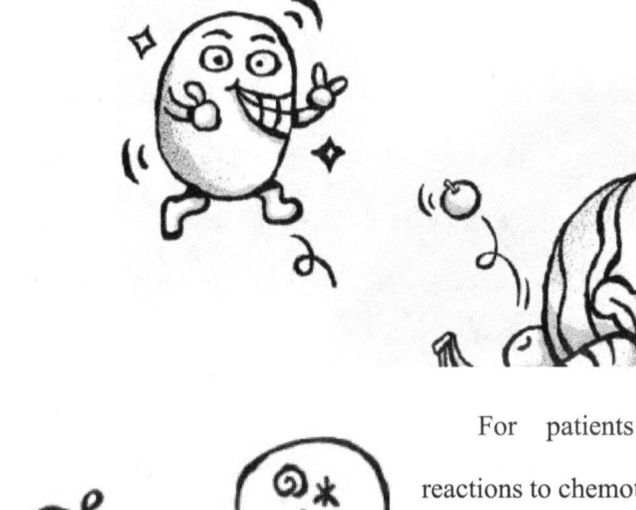

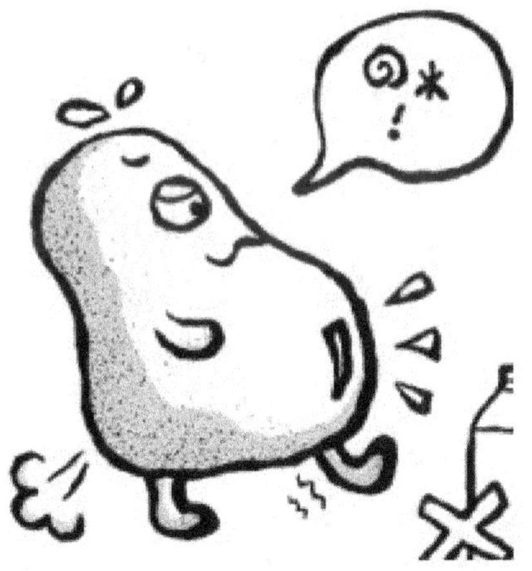

For patients with severe reactions to chemotherapy for liver cancer, some light and refreshing raw mixed cold dishes or some acidic foods with little or no oil can be used to stimulate the appetite, such as radish mixed with vinegar, cabbage heart mixed with vinegar, vegetarian salad, tremella mixed with celery, carrot shreds mixed with bean sprouts, and hawthorn cake mixed with duck pear. At the same time, simple, easy-to-use, and economical medicinal diet therapy can also be used, such as mushroom tofu soup, kelp sesame rice, and Hedyotis diffusa, coix seed and lotus seed porridge.

Adjust diet according to the type of tumor: patients with gastric cancer should avoid dog meat, smoked and roasted food, spicy seasonings, etc.; patients with esophageal cancer should avoid overheated drinks, alcohol, etc.; patients with liver cancer should avoid hard, fried, spicy food and alcohol; patients with breast cancer should eat less spicy food, avoid greasy food and alcohol; patients with liver cancer should avoid hard, fried, spicy food and alcohol; patients with intestinal cancer should avoid alcohol, processed food, and greasy food; patients with lung cancer should avoid alcohol and spicy food; patients with kidney cancer should eat less mutton, dog meat, salty food, alcohol and spicy food; patients with prostate cancer should avoid foods containing androgens, such as seahorses, deer antlers, leeks and leek flowers; patients with gallbladder cancer should avoid high-fat, alcohol and fried foods, and avoid overeating.

6. Ways to increase appetite during chemotherapy

(1) Change the recipe and cooking method.

(2) Medicinal food stimulates appetite and strengthens the spleen:

(i) Hawthorn diced meat: 100 g hawthorn, 1000 g lean pork (beef), 250 g vegetable oil, and appropriate amounts of mushrooms, ginger, onions, pepper, cooking wine, MSG, and sugar. First, cut the lean meat into slices, fry it in oil, then stew it with hawthorn seasoning and cook it until dry. It is both appetizing and anti-cancer.

(ii) Astragalus and Chinese Yam Soup: Use 30 g of Astragalus, add water and boil for half an hour, remove the residue, add 60 g of Chinese yam slices, boil for another 30 minutes, and add sugar (add honey for constipation). Take once a day in the morning and evening. It has the effects of invigorating Qi and promoting blood circulation, increasing appetite, and improving gastrointestinal absorption function.

(3) Eat more fresh vegetables and fruits with high vitamin content: This type of food can not only increase resistance, but also increase appetite. In the early postoperative period, patients can eat vegetable juice and a small amount of easily digestible fruit. The amount should not be too much each time, and patients should eat small meals frequently. After the gastrointestinal function has basically recovered, they can eat some light and refreshing raw mixed cold dishes and fruits, especially during chemotherapy and radiotherapy, which have a significant appetizing effect.

7. Common dietary care for toxic and side effects of chemotherapy

1. Anemia

(1) Eat appetizers to increase appetite. Eat more sweet and sour foods, and less bitter and spicy foods. Patients in chemotherapy are insensitive to sweet and sour tastes, but more sensitive to bitter tastes, so they should eat more sweet and sour foods. After chemotherapy, the body is weaker, so it is advisable to choose nutritious and easy-to-digest foods, such as soft food, porridge, bread, steamed buns, fish, eggs, chicken, soup, potatoes, bananas,

jam, etc.

(2) Selenium supplementation is essential. Selenium is an essential trace element for human health, often referred to as the "anti-cancer king" due to its potent protective properties. A large amount of survey data shows that the level of selenium content in food and soil in a region is directly related to the incidence of cancer. At present, the use of selenium as an auxiliary treatment in cancer treatment is very common. Selenium has a very strong antioxidant capacity. It can enhance the body's antioxidant capacity and prevent white blood cells from being killed by mistake.

(3) Eat more fresh vegetables and fruits with high vitamin content. These foods can not only increase resistance, but also increase appetite. Some patients believe that they should avoid eating raw and cold foods, but fruits and vegetables should be treated according to the situation. In the early postoperative period, patients can eat vegetable juice and a small amount of easily digestible fruit. The amount should not be too much each time, and they should eat small meals frequently. After the gastrointestinal function has basically recovered, they can eat some light and refreshing raw mixed cold dishes and fruits, especially during chemotherapy and radiotherapy, which have a significant appetizing effect.

2. Leukopenia after chemotherapy

Patients can start with strengthening the spleen, replenishing Qi and blood, and replenishing the kidney and essence in their diet. They should eat more yams, lentils, longan meat, jujubes, peanut kernels, black fungus, pig liver, turtle cooked with glutinous rice, pig bones, cattle bones, sheep bones, etc. If it is heart damage, manifested as arrhythmia, myocardial ischemia and chronic cardiomyopathy, etc., patients often feel chest tightness, panic, palpitations, fatigue and other symptoms, so they should eat more foods that have the effects of replenishing Qi, nourishing yin, widening the chest and regulating Qi, and promoting blood circulation and removing blood stasis. They can eat kudzu root powder, jujube, lily, wolfberry, citrus, hawthorn, ophiopogon, etc., which are beneficial to patients' bodies and minds.

In addition, drinking more green tea during chemotherapy can enhance the effectiveness of chemotherapy drugs in killing cancer cells without increasing toxic side effects.

After chemotherapy, patients should avoid eating greasy, spicy and irritating foods to avoid recurrence of symptoms.

In addition to dietary restrictions and nutritional supplements, patients should also protect their skin appropriately when their white blood cell count is low after chemotherapy, because the body's functions have not fully recovered at this time. In addition, many patients experience side effects after chemotherapy and feel very painful, so proper maintenance is necessary. Patients should keep their skin clean and dry, avoid using soap to scrub, and not apply irritating disinfectants such as alcohol and iodine. Avoid friction with hard and rough clothes. Avoid exposure to the sun, etc.

3. Hair loss

Patients should have a reasonable and scientific diet: nutritional supplements are necessary. Patients should take in more protein and calories to better deal with the side effects of chemotherapy and reduce the symptoms of hair loss. They should eat a light diet with high protein, easy to digest and absorb, and eat more fruits and vegetables rich in vitamins and inorganic salts. Eat less or no 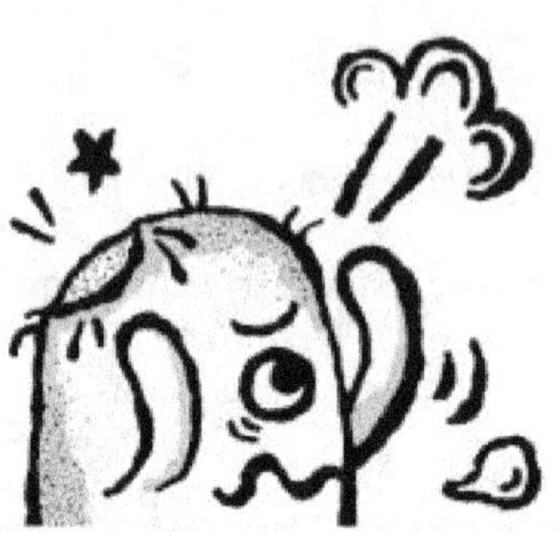 salted fish, pickles, bacon, cured meat and other foods containing nitrosamines. Avoid spicy and irritating foods and excessive drinking.

4. Nausea and vomiting

Patients should try to reduce their worries, because heavy mental burden and fear will induce or aggravate the occurrence of gastrointestinal reactions. They should gradually develop the habit of eating small meals and chewing slowly. Of course, although they should try to eat more, and there is no need to force themselves too much; try to eat some dry food and separate it from soup and drinks. It is best to eat a light liquid diet at the beginning, such as apple juice, orange juice, tea, etc., and avoid eating foods that are too sweet, too greasy, spicy, and smelly. In addition, food should not be overheated; cold food can be eaten to reduce the impact of odor; patients can take a proper walk before and after meals; eating small meals can reduce the amount of food eaten each time, increase the number of times, and reduce the burden of each meal. Try to make the food as varied as possible each time, or choose the food patients like to eat, which can promote appetite; eat less sweets, because sweets are easy to produce acid and gas; try not to eat greasy and fried food, because it is not easy to digest. If vomiting occurs while lying in bed, patients should lie on their side to prevent vomitus from being accidentally inhaled into the trachea. Rinse the mouth after vomiting and pay attention to the amount and nature of the vomitus. If necessary, keep a small amount of vomitus for testing. To ensure the daily food intake during chemotherapy, breakfast should be before 06:00 and dinner after 19:00. Prolonging the time difference between medication and eating can reduce reactions and promote food absorption.

5. Abdominal pain, diarrhea

When managing abdominal pain and diarrhea (common digestive tract symptoms), observe the following precautions: Pay attention to the nature and frequency of abdominal pain and diarrhea, because more serious toxic reactions can cause mucosal necrosis, shedding, and even perforation. If there are abnormalities, stool tests should be kept; soft food, less residue, low fiber, non-irritating food should be eaten, and foods that are easy to produce gas, such as sweet potatoes, corn, sorghum, beans, sugar, cabbage, cucumber,

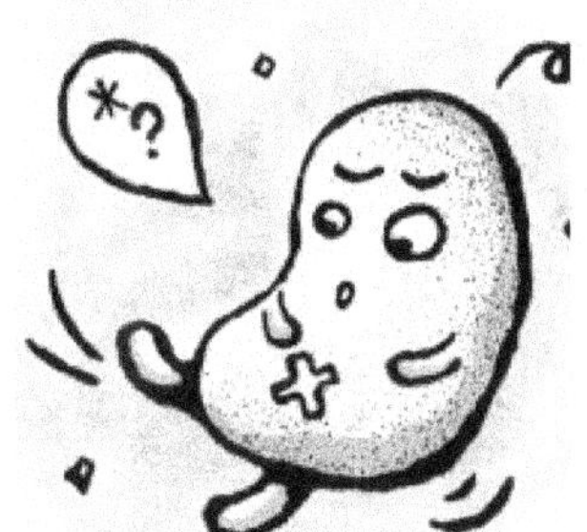

garlic, green pepper, and soda should not be consumed; pay attention to food hygiene to prevent gastrointestinal infections; drink about 3000 mL per day, to replenish the water lost by diarrhea and avoid water and electrolyte imbalance; keep the perineal skin clean, wash with warm water after defecation, and gently dry to avoid skin damage. If necessary, zinc oxide ointment can be applied locally to prevent corrosion of the skin around the anus.

6. Constipation

Constipation is often accompanied by symptoms such as loss of appetite and abdominal distension, which are mostly caused by a variety of reasons such as not eating enough, food that is too refined and lacks fiber, lack of activity, use of anesthetics, and mental stress. The following should be noted:

(1) Exercise appropriately. When clinically appropriate, patients are encouraged to engage in ambulation and light physical activity. If capable, they should gradually resume daily tasks and maintain self-care to the fullest extent possible. These activities provide dual benefits by: (i) stimulating gastrointestinal motility and (ii) improving psychological well-being through mood regulation, stress reduction, and enhanced quality of life.

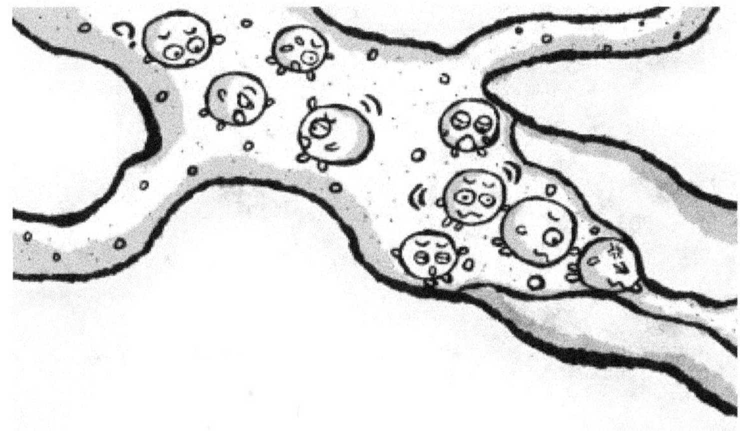

(2) Patients should maintain regular toilet visits according to their established bowel habits, even in the absence of an immediate urge. This timed defecation practice has been clinically shown to help prevent constipation by reinforcing natural gastrointestinal rhythms.

(3) The diet should contain an appropriate amount of fiber foods, such as celery and leeks, and eat more fresh vegetables, fruits and whole grains. People are encouraged to drink plenty of water, especially 200 mL of boiled water in the morning. It is best to drink cold water. If patients are not feeling well, they should drink slightly warmer water to effectively lubricate the intestines.

(4) If there is no bowel movement for 3 days, a laxative should be used. 30 mL of liquid paraffin can be taken orally 3 times a day. An enema can also be used.

(5) When the stool is dry, patients can use oil to perform a retention

enema to soften the stool and promote defecation.

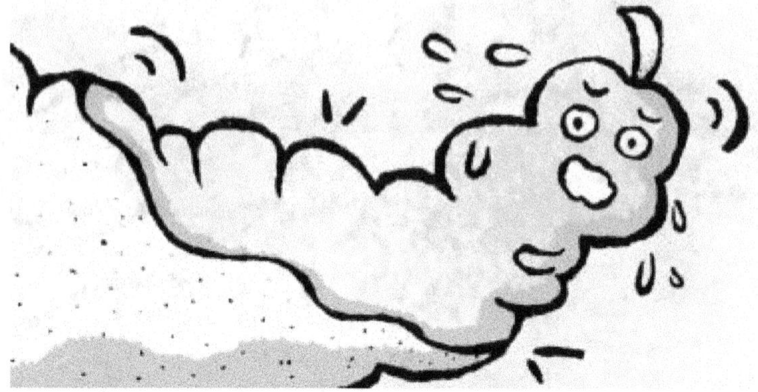

7. Oral ulcers

Patients should eat a non-irritating diet. The most acceptable foods are rice porridge, oatmeal porridge, vegetable puree, milk and egg paste, meat floss, ice cream, etc. If they can eat solid food and choose soft or well-cooked food. Avoid eating hard, coarse, cold, hot, and spicy food during chemotherapy.

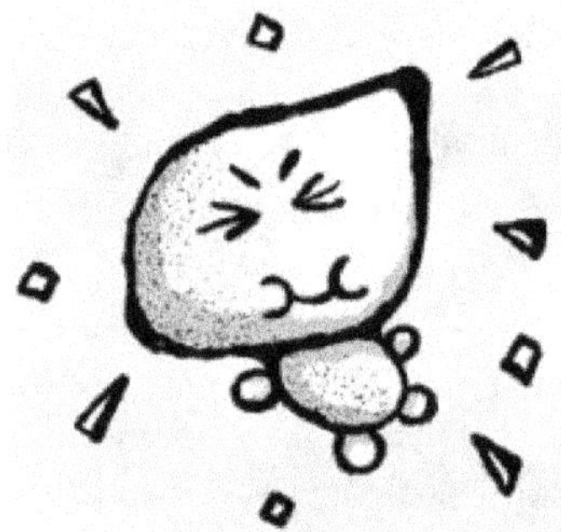

Part 5: To Defeat Cancer, Patients Must Have Confidence!

Cancer has become a prevalent global disease that significantly threatens human health. In recent years, with the influence of factors such as environment, dietary habits, and lifestyle changes, the incidence of cancer patients has increased year by year. The psychological burden of cancer patients has exceeded cardiovascular and cerebrovascular diseases and has become the number one cause of death. Because of this, the psychological burden of cancer patients is often heavy, which seriously affects the life quality of patients. It is particularly important to pay attention to the psychological problems of cancer patients.

1. Common mental health problems of cancer patients

1. Anxiety

Anxiety represents a complex psychological response to anticipated adverse outcomes. For cancer patients, the main causes of anxiety are the disability and pain that cancer may bring, threats to life, the pain that treatment may bring, economic losses, threats to the stability of family relationships, the weakening or loss of dignity, and the impact on the future. Anxiety has two main manifestations: one is acute anxiety disorder (panic attack) and the other is generalized anxiety, both of which can be accompanied by obvious symptoms of autonomic dysfunction.

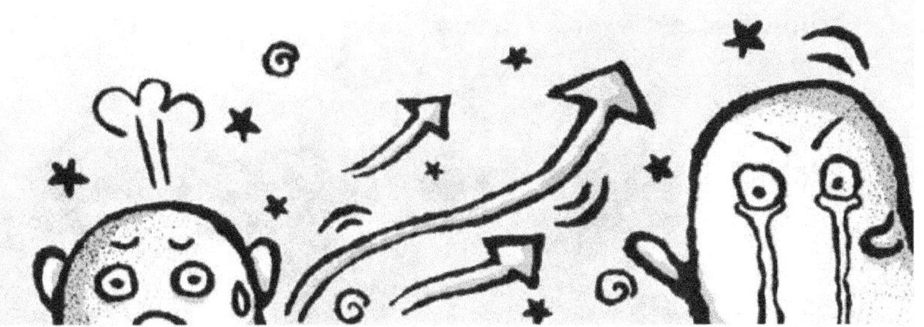

(1) Acute anxiety disorder (panic attack): The onset is acute and often occurs when waiting for a confirmed diagnosis or a preliminary diagnosis of cancer or when the condition changes suddenly.

(2) May be accompanied by the following autonomic nervous system symptoms: (i) palpitations; (ii) dyspnea; (iii)chest tightness, pressure or discomfort in the chest; (iv)throat obstruction or feeling of shortness of breath; (v) dizziness, lightheadedness or loss of balance; (vi) numbness in the hands and feet or abnormal sensation in the limbs; (vii) paroxysmal hot and cold sensations; (viii) sweating; (ix) syncope; and (x) tremors.

(3) Generalized anxiety disorder: Chronic or subacute onset, with the main symptoms being persistent mental and physical anxiety, such as sweating, tachycardia, dry mouth, facial flushing (or pale face), shortness of breath, frequent urination, urgency to urinate, and the urge to defecate. Severe anxiety can develop into fear.

2. Depression

Depression in cancer patients is characterized by persistent feelings of sadness, hopelessness, and emotional distress, frequently coexisting with anxiety. Patients are sad alone, avoid relatives, friends, and colleagues, and have suicidal intentions or actions (characteristics of depression). It can be observed that patients speak less, have low voices, move slowly, sit or lie in bed all day, and are too lazy to take

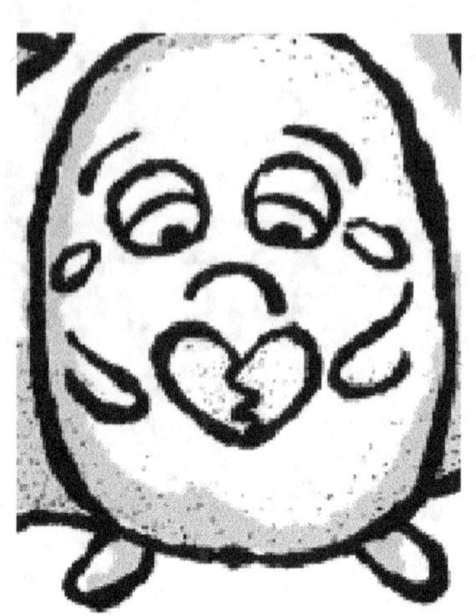

care of their daily lives. Depression often occurs in the late stage of the disease, and is often accompanied by physical disorders such as sleep disorders, decreased appetite, low libido, constipation, and weight loss. Consequently, clinicians must carefully differentiate depressive symptoms from tumor-related physical manifestations. Alarmingly, approximately 80% of cancer patients with depression remain undiagnosed or untreated.

3. Other psychiatric symptoms

(1) Irritability

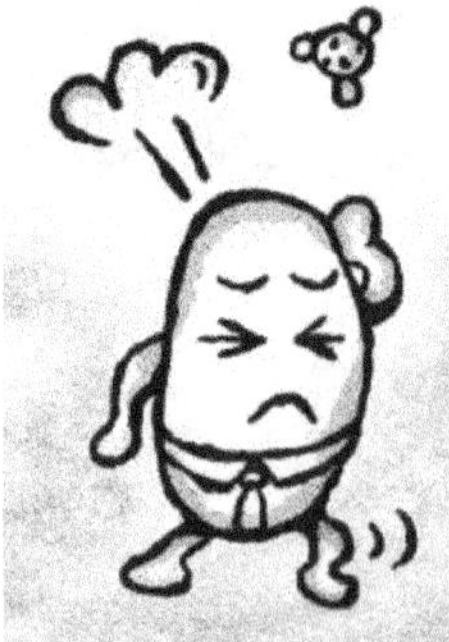

The hopelessness of treatment makes patients discouraged and irritable, which in turn causes greater mood fluctuations. They get excited, angry, indignant, sad, and cry over trivial matters. For example, if family members fail to visit on time or the food is not delicious, patients will get dissatisfied and find it hard to get along with. Patients feel that others are deliberately distancing them and even have a hostile attitude towards people around them. However, they may also be particularly affectionate to others and love to talk about their pain in the illness in order to win the sympathy of others.

(2) Loneliness

The main reasons for patients' loneliness are alienation from people around them, loneliness and helplessness, deprivation of social information and failure to meet the needs of their attachment to relatives.

(3) Feeling of helplessness

If patients believe that they have no control over their environment, they will feel helpless, which is a feeling of powerlessness and at a loss. Further generalization is depression. In connection with the feeling of helplessness, patients often have self-pity and bitterness, with countless grievances in their hearts that need to be vented, or are in a sleepwalking state, doing activities that are meaningless to others or themselves. It can be found that some patients sometimes say goodbye to themselves in front of the mirror, look back on the past, and feel sorry for themselves.

(4) Passive dependence

Cancer patients are more likely to receive care and attention from their family members and colleagues, becoming the center of attention. Patients themselves become passive, submissive, coquettish, dependent, emotionally fragile and even a little childish, and need help and care in every aspect of their lives.

(5) Suspicion

Suspicion is mostly a negative self-suggestion. It is a subjective guess, overly sensitive to everything around, thinking that doctors, family members, and colleagues are deliberately deceiving. In severe cases, paranoia or even persecution delusion, grandiose delusion, and hypochondria may occur.

(6) Projection reaction

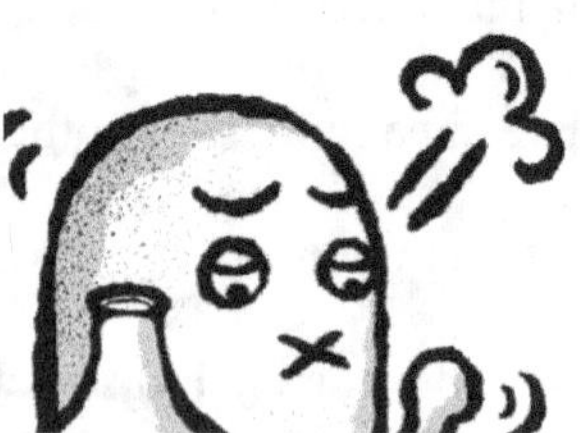

Introverted projection reactions are characterized by internalizing unacceptable thoughts, emotions, and impulses. Patients typically exhibit excessive self-blame, guilt over burdening family members with their illness, feelings of inferiority, social withdrawal, and in severe cases, suicidal ideation. This reaction pattern is more common in introverted individuals. Notably, prolonged introverted projection may unexpectedly transform into externalized anger when triggered by specific stimuli, leading to uncharacteristic outbursts directed at caregivers or family members.

Extroverted projection reactions are characterized by externalizing blame, where patients disproportionately attribute problems to external circumstances or others while minimizing personal responsibility. These patients often make excessive demands regarding treatment, frequently complain about inadequate care from family members, and react angrily to minor issues, potentially straining therapeutic and personal relationships. When unable to direct their frustration outward, extroverted projectors may shift to self-destructive behaviors (including treatment refusal) or develop secondary depressive symptoms, demonstrating the dynamic nature of these psychological responses.

(7) Memory impairment

In the early stages, the disease often presents with recent memory loss or amnesia, and the memory of past experiences cannot be reproduced, or even distorted. However, memory can be relatively well maintained in time, but disorientation often occurs as the disease progresses.

(8) Emotional disorders

Indifference to external things, dull expression, lack of initiative. In addition, there may be crying and laughing for no reason, emotional instability, fidgeting, irritability, anxiety, depression or abnormal euphoria.

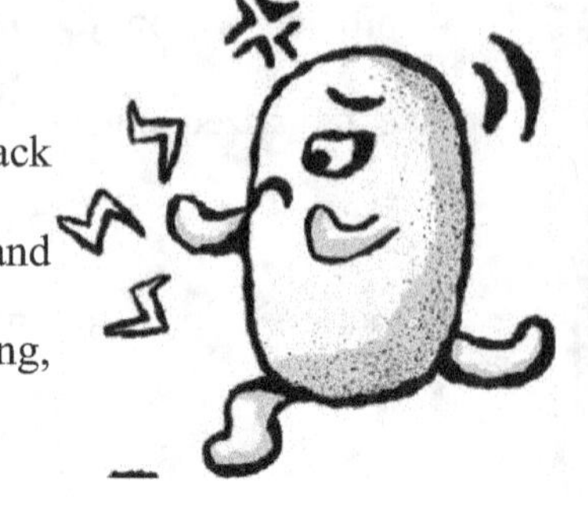

(9) Perceptual impairment

Auditory hallucinations are more common, but there may also be visual, olfactory and tactile hallucinations. Sometimes, sensory hypersensitivity or loss of sensation and perceptual complex disorders can be seen.

(10) Delirium

This condition is characterized by fluctuating levels of consciousness and diurnal variation in disorientation, typically milder in the morning and worsening in the evening. Patients often have psychomotor agitation, such as restlessness, constant twisting of the body, or carphology. They often do not answer questions or answer irrelevant questions. Sometimes they mumble to themselves and their thoughts are incoherent. They may also have hallucinations or delusions.

(11) Hallucination state

A large number of auditory and visual hallucinations suddenly occur without obvious disturbance of consciousness. The contents are mostly horrific, so there are horrific expressions and escape reactions. Patients who are receiving or preparing to receive chemotherapy are often prone to olfactory and gustatory hallucinations.

(12) Acute dementia

Patients are conscious, but have obvious cognitive and thinking disorders, memory loss, reduced calculation and comprehension abilities, and even worse judgment and reasoning abilities. For example, he/she does not recognize his/her relatives, cannot name common things, and speaks in a childish and ridiculous manner. After a period of time, he/she can fully recover to normal.

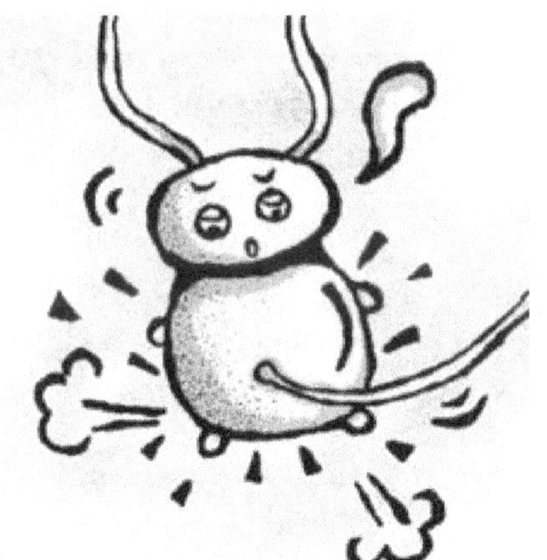

(13) Wandering

Patients are in a state of confusion and wander aimlessly, or move aimlessly from one place to another, but can avoid obstacles or dangers. Examination shows that patients have a blank expression. It usually lasts for a few hours to a few days, and can suddenly wake up, completely forgetting the whole process or only having scattered fragments of memory.

(14) Stupor-like state

Common in severe depressive episodes, patients first feel heaviness in the limbs, and develop psychomotor inhibition syndrome under clear and normal consciousness. In mild cases, speech and movement are significantly reduced, or slow and sluggish, sitting, standing or lying in bed motionless, expressionless, silent and unresponsive to various stimuli. During the examination, it can be found that

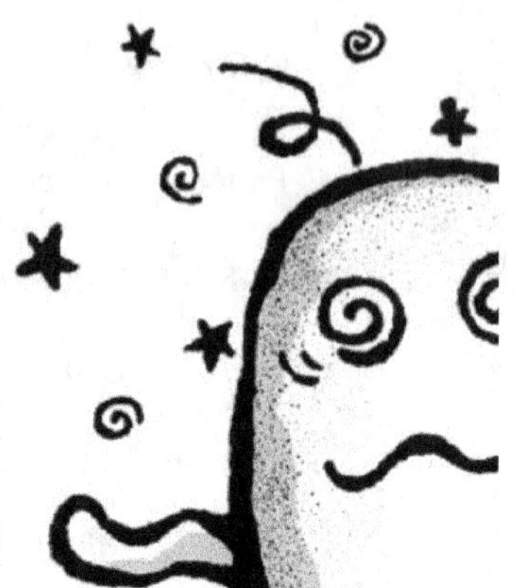

patients' eyes track moving objects, or stare at the examiner. If they are asked patiently, a weak answer can often be obtained, or they will nod or shake their heads to indicate, and sometimes tears can be seen in the corners of their eyes, which is completely different from a coma. Reactive stupor in cancer patients is generally short-lived and often resolves naturally.

(15) Silence

In a state of clear consciousness, patients remain silent, do not answer any questions verbally, and do not speak, but sometimes can express their opinions through gestures, writing or facial expressions. Unlike stupor, patients have no motor inhibition. Mutism can be caused by compression of intracranial tumors, which should be carefully identified.

(16) Manic-like reactions

The most characteristic clinical manifestations include psychomotor agitation, flight of ideas, and mood elevation. Psychomotor excitement, marked by significantly increased speech and motor activity, may present as either coordinated (when aligned with thoughts and emotions) or uncoordinated. In cancer patients, this typically manifests as emotional excitement with heightened verbal output and movement, often featuring comprehensible speech content related to psychological factors or personal experiences. Patients may appear euphoric, irritable, or grandiose, frequently attempting to direct other patients' activities.

Patients experiencing flight of ideas demonstrate accelerated thought processes, rapidly generating new concepts with superficially rich content. While their thinking maintains some purpose, they frequently shift topics in response to environmental stimuli, preventing coherent thought completion. They often exhibit pressured speech, subjectively feeling exceptionally quick-witted and capable of effortless eloquence. Elevated mood presents as unwarranted cheerfulness, exaggerated

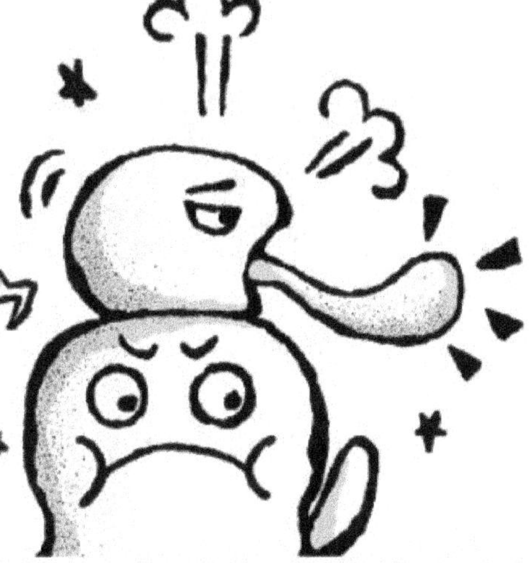

optimism (as if unaffected by cancer), and inflated self-confidence with interests in all matters. However, this emotional state often proves labile, with sudden shifts to sadness or anger triggered by minor stimuli.

(17) Identity issues

Patients with mental problems such as anxiety and depression often do not admit that they have psychological abnormalities. They appear to be calm and indifferent, and sometimes they are uncooperative with medical staff.

(18) Suicide

Having thoughts of suicide but not taking action is called suicidal ideation; if one is ready to take action, it is called a suicide attempt; intentionally taking actions that are not enough to cause death, or just making a suicidal appearance with the intention of warning, threatening or asking for help, is called a suicidal gesture, which can sometimes also lead to death.

2. Why do these psychological problems exist?

There are many factors that affect the mental and psychological problems of cancer patients, including factors related to cancer disease and treatment, general factors, and social and psychological factors.

1. Factors related to cancer disease and treatment

(1) Pain: Many cancer patients believe that pain means disease progression and death. If pain is not properly controlled, anxiety and

depression will become more obvious.

(i) Tumor location: The incidence of depression varies with different tumors. The treatment of breast cancer, head and neck cancer, rectal cancer, and penile cancer may cause image damage and produce special psychological problems.

(ii) Physical fitness: Patients with poor scores are higher than those with good scores.

(2) Surgical treatment: The incidence of moderate psychological disorders, especially depression, in patients with colorectal cancer who underwent colostomy was significantly higher than that in patients who retained the anus.

(i) Chemotherapy: Chemotherapy is more likely to cause depression than surgery, affecting patients' life quality. Patients who relapse after treatment feel more desperate.

(ii) Radiotherapy: Compared with chemotherapy, the psychological reaction caused by radiotherapy is milder and lasts for a shorter time.

2. General and socio-psychological factors

(1) Age: Children have a smaller psychological reaction to the disease. Middle-aged people have a heavy responsibility and react more to the disease. Due to their age, the elderly usually react less to tumors than young people. However, most data show that depression in cancer patients is not related to

age.

(2) Gender and marriage: There are more female patients than male ones suffering from psychological problems. There is a clear correlation between marriage and depression, and divorced and separated people are more likely to suffer from depression.

(3) Social status: People with high social status have stronger psychological reactions than those with low social status; people who live a happy and loved life have stronger psychological reactions than those who live a difficult and hard life.

(4) Educational level: People with higher education levels have a better understanding of diseases and have stronger psychological reactions. Among people with higher education levels, the psychological pressure on patients and medical staff is particularly obvious.

(5) Economic income: Generally speaking, people with high economic income have fewer worries and their psychological reactions may be milder, but the opposite may also be true.

(6) Personality traits: Patients' cognition and response to cancer are based on their own personality traits.

(7) Religious beliefs: Devout believers may view cancer as a necessary tribulation on the way to heaven and thus show less mental pain. They may also view cancer as a retribution for past sins and suffer greatly from mental

torture.

(8) Illness experience: People who are often ill have better tolerance and may have less psychological pressure. On the other hand, people who have always been healthy are less mentally prepared and react more strongly.

(9) Social support: Studies on cancer patients have shown that although social support cannot improve patients' physical symptoms, it can significantly improve their psychological state. The family's understanding and attitude towards the tumor, and the quality of the relationship with relatives, colleagues, and neighbors can sometimes significantly affect patients' mood.

3. What to do when facing these psychological problems?

(1) Transform disease perceptions: The need for survival is the strongest need of every cancer patient. Nurses should tirelessly strengthen health knowledge guidance for patients and their family, and provide patients with timely information such as the nature and extent of the disease, the advantages and disadvantages of possible treatment options, and precautions during treatment, so as to increase patients' sense of control over the disease, change their misconceptions about cancer, and encourage them to face the challenges of the disease and the discomfort of treatment with a positive attitude.

(2) Improve patients' coping abilities: Once patients are diagnosed with

cancer, they are under threat of death, and different coping skills can achieve different coping effects for different patients. The most appropriate coping skills for cancer are to face and accept reality directly, solve problems in a timely manner, and live a positive life.

(3) Assist in establishing good interpersonal relationships: Good interpersonal relationships and extensive social support are important links in alleviating negative emotions and improving the body's immunity. Strengthening interpersonal intimacy can help patients reduce or forget the pain caused by the disease, and can help them gain strength to fight the disease. At the same time, cancer patients not only need sympathy, care and concern, but also understanding and respect. Help them restore the original social support system destroyed by cancer, so that they can receive the love and help of fellow patients, and the comfort and closeness of relatives and friends.

(4) Increase patients' sense of security: Cancer patients need to be protected and hope to have a comfortable, quiet, well-ventilated, and sunny environment. They also need medical staff with superb medical skills, a kind attitude, and dedication to treat them.

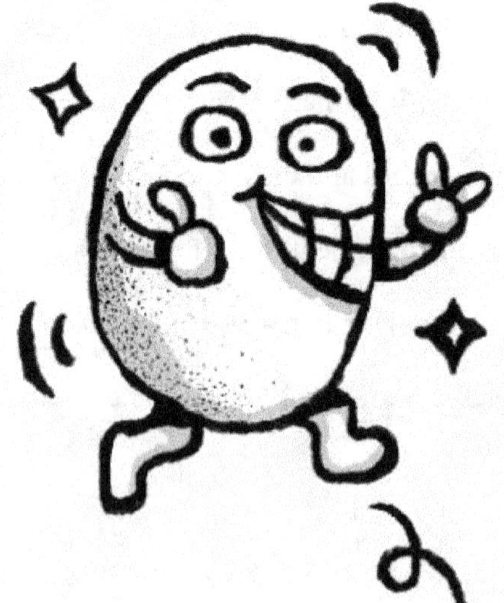

4. Nursing measures for the psychological status of patients in the early, middle and late stages

1. Protective care

Protective care requires strict adherence to confidentiality protocols. Protective measures should be taken for patients who are unaware of the disease, those who have anxiety and fear reactions to the disease, and those who are emotionally fragile to prevent them from losing self-control due to excessive psychological burden. Explain the harm of tumors and the benefits of treatment so that patients can actively cooperate with treatment. Understand the psychological dynamics of patients and provide timely and effective information for personalized care.

2. Nursing during treatment

Psychological factors play a very important role in people's diseases and health. Pay attention not only to the effect of drug treatment, but to the therapeutic effect of non-drug psychological nursing intervention. Good psychological counseling should be provided for patients at all stages.

(1) Before treatment: Timely introduce chemotherapy precautions and related matters that require cooperation, explain possible adverse reactions during treatment, preventive measures, and avoid patients giving up treatment due to adverse reactions. This is an important part of psychological care for malignant tumors that cannot be ignored.

(2) During treatment: During chemotherapy, according to patients' interests and hobbies, choose appropriate distraction methods, such as music therapy, to divert their attention and create a new environment to relieve their realistic pressure, thereby reducing their discomfort. During chemotherapy, keep the infusion unobstructed to prevent fluid extravasation, communicate and talk with them more, avoid using a didactic tone, do not use false and inappropriate comfort, avoid explanations that are not very targeted, and avoid hasty conclusions or answers, so as to reduce patients' doubts and enable them to successfully complete each stage of chemotherapy.

(3) After treatment: After chemotherapy, timely resumption of some work can help patients realize their own value and their role in society, thus regaining their spirits. Reasonable and correct psychological nursing intervention measures are not only beneficial to the treatment effect of cancer patients, but also can greatly improve the life quality of patients.

3. Cancer pain care

Pain is one of the common symptoms of patients with advanced tumors, especially persistent and difficult-to-control pain. This chronic pain significantly compromises patients' quality of life, often causing profound suffering and distress. Avoid using negative language, which can easily make patients pessimistic and disappointed and aggravate their condition. Thoughtfulness, caring, and comforting language often have an effect that drugs cannot achieve. Understanding patients' pain, listening carefully to their story, affirming their tolerance to pain, and psychologically alleviating anxiety and uneasiness are all positive for relieving pain.

4. End-of-life care

Cancer patients often experience rapid disease progression. Most patients are still conscious before clinical death. Faced with the fact that they are about to end their lives, their psychological activities are complex and their bodies and minds are in great pain. Hospice care is a positive and comprehensive care for patients who have lost hope of recovery and are about to end their lives. Various effective measures can be taken: (i) Give patients more encouragement and comfort, communicate with them emotionally, listen to them patiently, speak more positively, and stimulate their potential survival consciousness; (ii) Pay attention to patients' will and small wishes, try to meet their requirements in life care, stabilize their emotions, and maximize the their physical, psychological, and social needs; (iii) When the condition deteriorates rapidly and various treatments fail, patients' late psychological performance is drastic, and accidents must be prevented; (iv) Reduce patients' physical and psychological pain and let them spend the rest of their life in peace.

Part 6: Understanding Cancer Pain

Pain is one of the most prevalent clinical manifestations of cancer patients. According to statistics from the WHO, there are approximately 6 million new cancer cases worldwide each year, and approximately 4 million patients suffer from cancer pain every day, of which 50% to 80% do not receive satisfactory relief. Among advanced-stage patients, 60-90% report severe pain, with roughly 25% dying without obtaining sufficient relief from their intense pain symptoms.

1. What is cancer pain?

Cancer pain results from the transmission of pain signals from affected areas to the central nervous system, requiring intervention for relief. In advanced cancer patients, this pain represents a primary source of significant distress. Pain comprises two key components: pain perception (the conscious awareness of pain) and pain response (the body's reaction). Pain perception serves as a critical warning system, alerting to bodily harm while often triggering intense emotional reactions including anxiety, fear, and distress.

The pain response is mediated through three primary reflex systems: (1) somatic-motor reflexes (manifested as clenched fists or muscle spasms); (2) autonomic-visceral reflexes (e.g., increased respiration, elevated blood pressure, pupillary dilation, and sweating); and (3) neuro-psychiatric reflexes (e.g., anxiety and other psychological responses). These complex physiological and emotional reactions underscore the multifaceted nature of cancer pain and its significant impact on patient wellbeing.

2. How does cancer pain occur?

1. Physical factors

(1) Tumor-related pain: It can be divided into direct and indirect pain.

Pain directly caused by the tumor:

(i) Tissue destruction: When the tumor invades the pleura, peritoneum or nerves, such as bone metastasis, bone tumors causing bone pain. Lung cancer invading the pleura can cause chest pain.

(ii) Compression: Brain tumors can cause headaches and cranial neuralgia. Metastasis of nasopharyngeal carcinoma to the neck can cause compression and neck, shoulder, and arm pain. Compression of retroperitoneal tumors can cause waist and abdominal pain.

(iii) Blockage: When a hollow organ is obstructed by a tumor, discomfort and cramps may occur. Complete obstruction can lead to severe colic, as seen in gastric, intestinal, or pancreatic cancers. In addition, when breast cancer metastasizes to the axillary lymph nodes, it can compress the lymph and blood vessels in the axillary area and cause swelling and pain in the

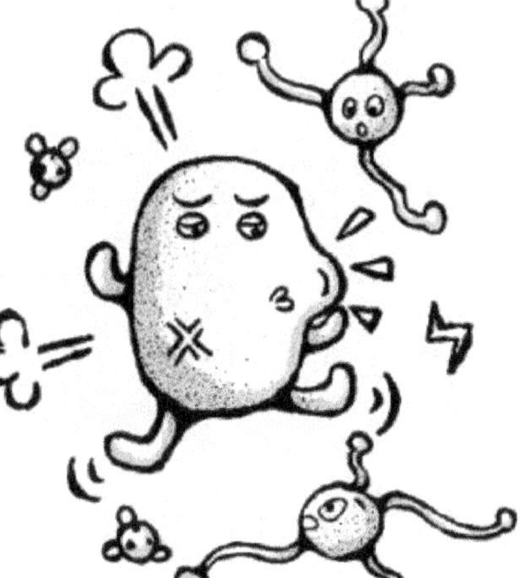

affected arm.

(iv) Tension: When the primary and liver metastatic tumors grow rapidly, the liver capsule is overstretched and tightened, which may cause severe distension and pain in the right upper abdomen.

(v) Tumor ulceration: If it does not heal for a long time and infection occurs, it may cause severe pain.

(2) Anti-tumor treatment-related pain occurs in about 8.2% of cases and is a common complication of cancer therapy. Examples include: (i) Post-radiotherapy: local damage, peripheral nerve damage fibrosis, radiation neuritis, stomatitis, dermatitis, radiation osteonecrosis, etc. (ii) Post-chemotherapy/radiotherapy herpes zoster may occur and cause pain. (iii) after chemotherapy: chemotherapy drugs leak out of blood vessels and cause tissue necrosis, chemotherapy-induced thrombotic phlebitis, an toxic peripheral neuritis. Damage to the axillary lymphatic system during radical mastectomy can cause swelling and pain in the arm. (iv) after surgery, incision scars, nerve damage, and phantom limb pain.

(3) Non-tumor pain: accounting for about 7.2%. Clinically, a small number of cancer patients may experience pain that is not related to the tumor, such as pain in bones and joints, aneurysms, and diabetic peripheral neuropathy.

2. Social and psychological factors

Caused by fear, anxiety, depression, anger, loneliness and other factors.

3. The impact of cancer pain

(1) Impact on mental health: Acute pain can cause patients to become hyperactive, anxious, irritable, and unable to sleep or eat. Long-term chronic pain can cause depression.

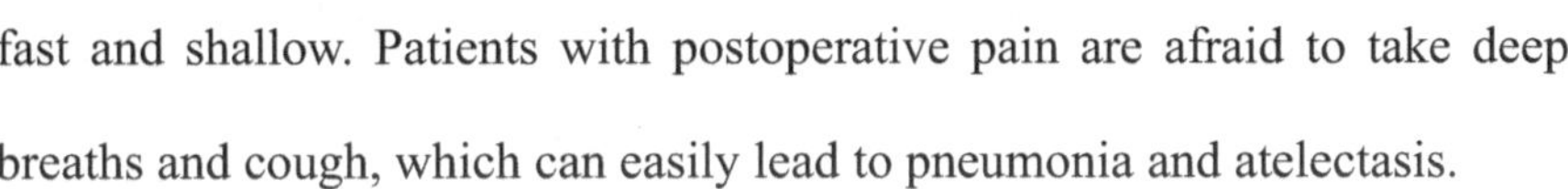

(2) Impact on the respiratory system: When the pain is severe, the breathing is fast and shallow. Patients with postoperative pain are afraid to take deep breaths and cough, which can easily lead to pneumonia and atelectasis.

(3) Impact on the cardiovascular system: Superficial pain has an excitatory effect on the circulation, leading to increased blood pressure and heart rate. In contrast, deep pain has an inhibitory effect, resulting in low blood pressure, a slow pulse, and in severe cases, may even cause shock.

(4) Impact on the digestive system: Chronic pain often causes nausea, vomiting, loss of appetite, and digestive dysfunction.

(5) Impact on the neuroendocrine system: Pain puts the body in a state of stress, causing abnormal secretion of multiple hormones in the body, resulting in the body consuming huge amounts of energy.

(6) Impact on the immune system: Pain can cause a decline in immune function, which is not conducive to the prevention or treatment, as well as the control of tumor spread.

(7) Impact on coagulation function: Pain puts the body in a hypercoagulable state. In addition, patients are afraid to turn over or get out of bed due to pain, which can easily lead to the formation of deep vein thrombosis in the lower extremities.

Part 7: Cancer Pain Treatment

1. Goals of cancer pain treatment

(1) Relieve the pain continuously and effectively.

(2) Avoid or reduce the adverse reactions of analgesics.

(3) Minimize the psychological and mental burden of pain and treatment on patients.

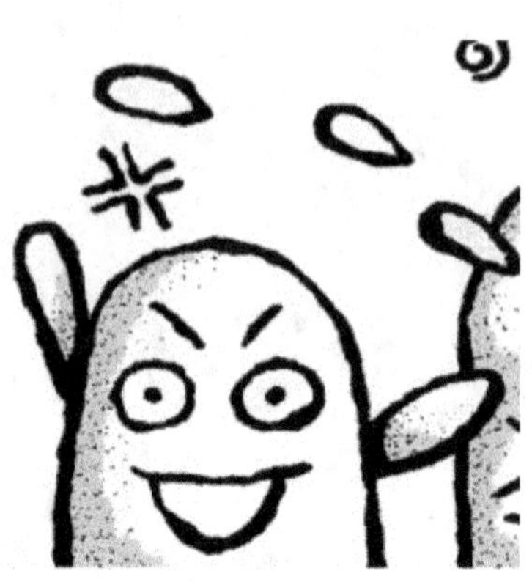

(4) Maximize the life quality of cancer pain patients.

2. Treatment according to the cause of cancer pain

The primary etiologies of cancer-related pain include both the malignancy itself and its associated complications. Various anti-cancer therapies - including palliative surgery, radiotherapy, and chemotherapy - can provide varying degrees of pain relief for cancer patients.

(1) Radiotherapy Radiation therapy

Referred to as radiation therapy, it plays an important role in cancer pain and other tumor patients. A large amount of data and successful clinical experience have confirmed that it has good effects and high value in the treatment of bone metastasis, dura mater tumors, and brain metastasis.

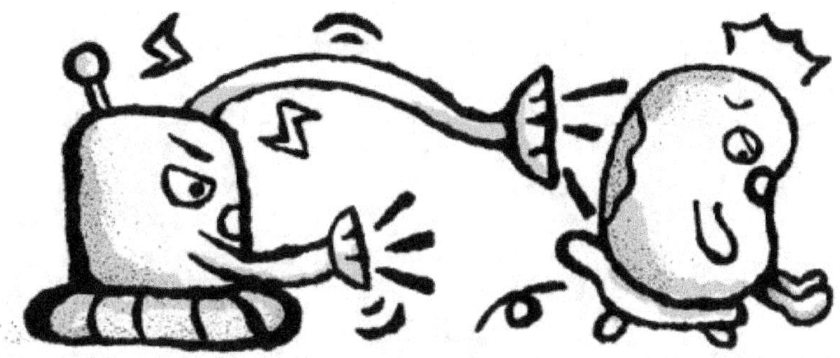

(2) Chemotherapy

Chemotherapy is a good method with a specific analgesic effect. Tumor shrinkage after chemotherapy is correlated with pain relief.

(3) Palliative surgery

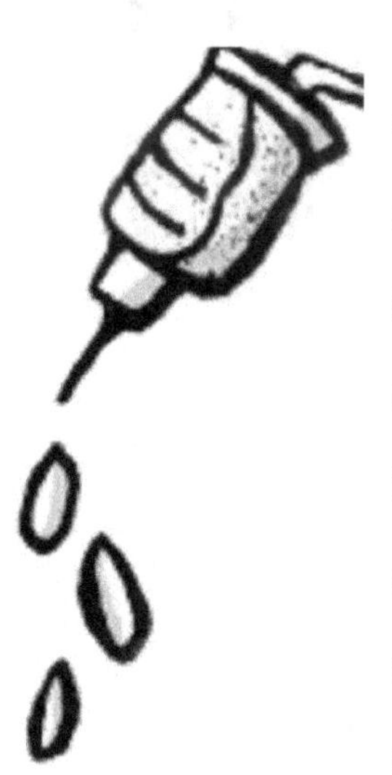

Surgery can relieve pain caused by certain diseases, especially intestinal obstruction, unstable bone structure and nerve compression. Surgery to control cancer pain is a destructive method. Neurolysis, percutaneous or open anterior lateral column myelotomy, body-directed central nerve cauterization, etc., are also methods of relieving cancer pain. However, it must be performed by experienced neurosurgeons.

3. Cancer pain medication

Clinically, drugs are the main treatment for cancer pain. Therefore, it is necessary to comprehensively, accurately and timely assess the duration, degree, location, nature, persistence and discontinuity of pain, pain treatment history, and the impact of pain on patients and their families.

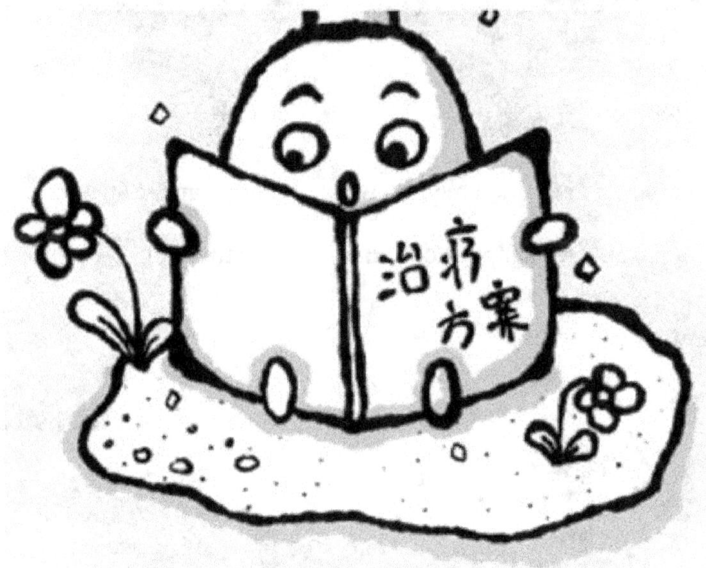

1. General principles of drug treatment for cancer pain

Oral medication for first choice: Regular oral administration of morphine has become the mainstay of treatment for chronic cancer pain.

Individualization principle: select the dosage that suits each individual, that is, implement individualization. The dosage of analgesics varies from person to person, and the effective analgesic dosage varies greatly among different patients.

Treatment of insomnia: The pain usually worsens at night, affecting the sleep of patients undergoing chemotherapy and radiotherapy. If this continues for a long time, it will lead to neurasthenia in patients. The dose of morphine should be increased at night to prolong the analgesia time so that patients can sleep well.

Dealing with side effects: Strong opioids often cause side effects such as constipation, nausea, and vomiting, which require treatment with antiemetics and laxatives. Long-term oral opioids rarely cause respiratory depression that requires treatment.

Observation of the effects: Regardless of the analgesic used, the therapeutic effects and side effects must be observed in detail.

2. Use medication correctly

According to the pain assessment results, analgesics are given according to the doctors' instructions and the three-step analgesia principle. The basic principles to be followed when administering analgesics are:

(1) Oral administration: It is the main and preferred non-invasive route of administration. The reasons are: (i) simple, economical, and easy to accept; (ii) stable blood drug concentration; (iii) as effective as intravenous injection; (iv) easier to adjust the dosage and more autonomous; (v) less addictive and less likely to cause drug resistance.

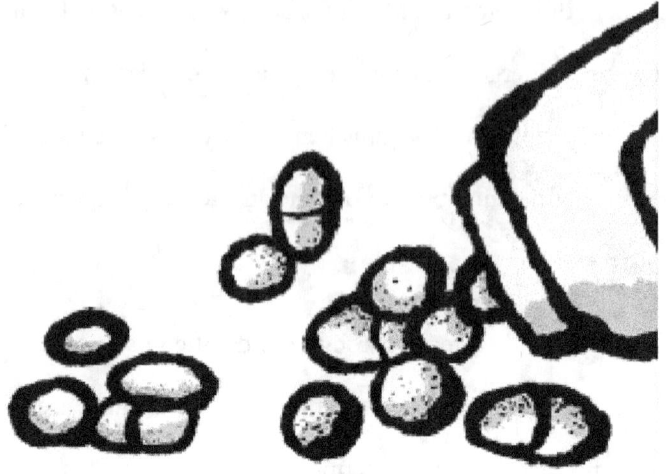

(2) Administration in a step-by-step manner: Increase the dosage gradually according to the principle of from weak to strong, from small to large, and from little to much. Do not wait until patients need it before using it. Take the medicine regularly and carefully observe the efficacy and side effects.

(3) Administration on time: Strictly control the half-life of analgesics and administer medication regularly, rather than administering medication on demand, to ensure continuous pain relief.

(4) Individualized medication: The development of an individualized analgesic regimen should be based on each patient's clinical condition and response to cancer pain medication. The sensitivity to anesthetic drugs varies greatly from person to person, so there is no standard dosage for opioids. The dose that can relieve pain and minimize side effects is the optimal dose.

(5) Specific details: Patients using painkillers should be closely monitored, their pain relief and body response should be closely observed, attention should be paid to the interactions of combined drug use, and necessary measures should be taken in a timely manner to minimize adverse drug reactions, improve the effectiveness of analgesic treatment, and ultimately improve patient quality of life.

4. Observation and nursing care of common adverse reactions of analgesics

1. Non-opioid adverse reactions

(1) Blood system: It causes platelet aggregation, i.e., the disaggregation of agglutinated platelets. Clinically, it can cause bleeding.

(2) Gastrointestinal reactions: Long-term use may cause indigestion, nausea, diarrhea, constipation, and abdominal distension. Long-term use of large doses may cause gastrointestinal bleeding or ulcers.

(3) Effects on the kidneys: Prostaglandins regulate renal blood flow, water and sodium balance, etc.

(4) Effects on liver function: Long-term use can cause toxic changes in the liver, renal damage and myocardial ischemia.

2. Common adverse reactions of opioids and their treatment

(1) Constipation: The most common and often treatment-limiting side

effect. Prevention: drink plenty of water, eat more fiber-containing foods, exercise appropriately, and take laxatives preventively. Treatment: assess the cause and degree of constipation, select laxatives according to the degree of constipation, and perform an enema if necessary.

(2) Nausea and vomiting: Differential diagnosis should exclude other causes such as constipation, brain metastasis, chemotherapy, radiotherapy, and hypercalcemia. Generally, in the early stage of medication, most of them are relieved within 4 to 7 days, and then gradually alleviated and completely disappeared. Prevention and treatment: For the first use, it is best to use antiemetic drugs for prevention within the first week. Metoclopramide is commonly used, three times a day, half an hour before meals. If the symptoms persist for more than one week and other causes are excluded, the dosage of opioids should be reduced or the medicine should be changed, or other routes of administration should be used.

(3) Sedation: Chronic pain often leads to insomnia, which may persist even after achieving adequate pain control. During the initial phase of opioid therapy, when the drug dose is significantly increased. Prevention: The initial dose should not be too high. The elderly should be especially careful in titrating the dose. If patients are obviously over-sedated, the dose of opioids should be reduced. If the degree of sedation continues to worsen, patients' consciousness and breathing should be closely observed.

(4) Urinary retention: Prevention: Avoid using sedatives at the same

time, and urinate regularly (e.g., urinate every 4 hours). Treatment: Inducing spontaneous urination (inducing water, pouring hot water into the perineum, and gently massaging the bladder area). If it is still ineffective, consider catheterization.

(5) Central nervous system toxicity: Patients who use pethidine for a long time are at risk of central nervous system toxicity. Symptoms include tremors, tremors, convulsions, and epileptic seizures. Therefore, pethidine is only used for short-term analgesia and is not suitable for chronic pain.

5. Non-drug pain relief care

1. Attention distraction

Attention distraction—shifting focus from pain to other stimuli—can enhance pain relief. Techniques include social interaction (e.g., conversation), engaging activities (e.g., playing cards or chess), or relaxation methods such as sitting comfortably, closing one's eyes while recalling pleasant memories, or listening to uplifting music. These interventions, practiced for 20-minute sessions, can amplify analgesic effects.

2. Relaxation

Allow patients to relax their whole bodies, such as closing their eyes, counting numbers, yawning, lying flat with knees and hips bent, relaxing abdominal muscles, and allowing them to take deep breath, inhale through the nose, and then exhale slowly with the mouth open, so as to relax their whole bodies, block or weaken the pain response, and achieve the purpose of pain relief.

3. Physical methods

Includes hot and cold compresses, massage, activity, immobilization, and subcutaneous electrical nerve stimulation.

4. Diet therapy

Studies have found that for patients with advanced liver cancer and ascites, eating fresh grapes or raisins; raw and cold foods, such as fruits and vegetables; or a mixed diet of 1/4 cereals, yogurt, eggs, animal liver, etc., and 3/4 fruits and vegetables, these dietary therapies can relieve cancer pain.

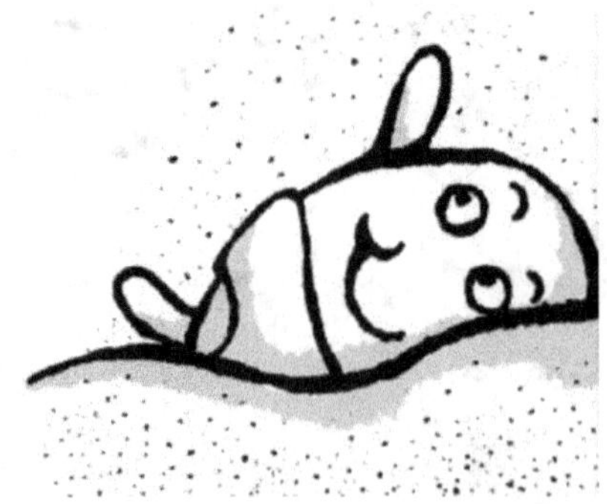

6. Psychological care

1. Catharsis

Take the initiative to care for patients warmly, spend time with them, listen to their concerns with empathy, and reassure them that they are not alone in their struggle. This helps ease their sense of isolation and reminds them that others understand and support them.

2. Comforting

Comforting should be just right, emphasizing the hopeful aspects without being too optimistic, and helping patients analyze the responsiveness of pain.

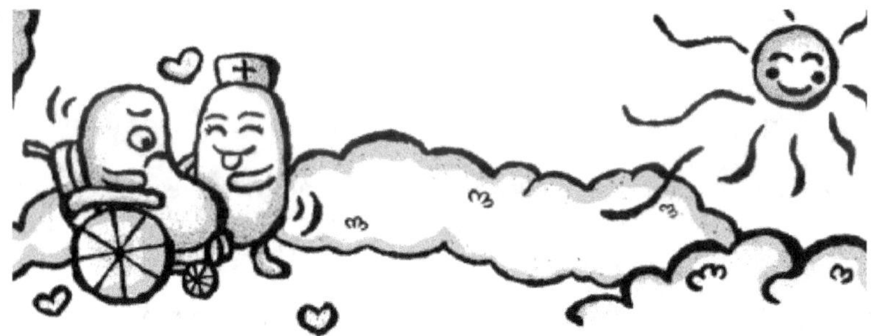

3. Suggestion therapy

Let patients realize that pain is a protective reaction of the body in its fight against the disease, which means that the body is in a state of adjustment and the pain is temporary. As long as the disease is defeated, the pain will naturally disappear. Encourage patients to increase their confidence.

4. Psychological care for family members

The care from family members is very important to patients. Family members should give comfort, encouragement and support to patients, so that patients can get rid of the fear and terror of pain mentally and increase their hope for life.

7. Health Education

(1) Patients should be encouraged to actively report their pain levels. Most cancer-related pain can be effectively managed through medication when taken as prescribed under physician supervision. Pain management is an essential component of comprehensive cancer care. Patients should strictly adhere to their prescribed medication regimen without self-adjusting dosages or schedules, as unrelieved pain may hinder recovery and negatively impact overall well-being.

(2) Morphine and similar opioids are standard medications for managing cancer pain, with addiction being exceptionally rare when used appropriately 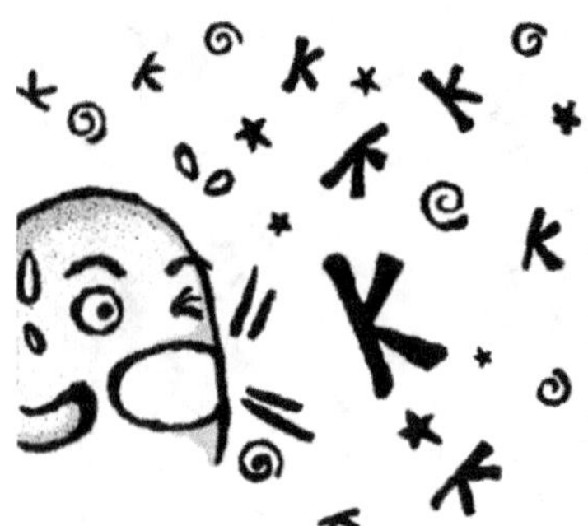 for pain control. These medications must be stored securely under proper conditions. During treatment, patients require close monitoring for both therapeutic effects and potential adverse reactions, with ongoing communication between healthcare providers and patients to optimize pain management strategies. Regular follow-up visits and continuous treatment monitoring are essential components of effective pain control.

Part 8: Common Misunderstandings of Cancer Pain Treatment

There are many misunderstandings of cancer pain treatment, which seriously affect cancer pain control and the life quality of patients.

Misunderstanding 1: If patients have cancer, patients will definitely feel pain, and enduring pain is a virtue.

This is a misconception. Freedom from pain is a fundamental human right. Pain can seriously reduce a person's quality of life, increase anxiety, depression, and world-weariness. Current medical technology can be used to control cancer pain very well. Pain needs to 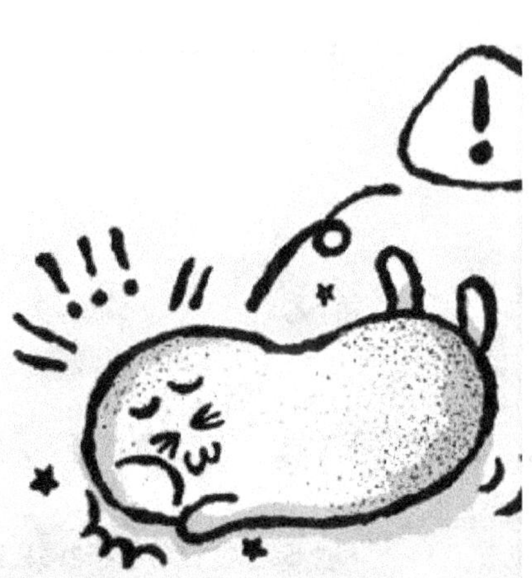 be treated, and it must be standardized treatment.

Misunderstanding 2: Three-step medication is to divide the drugs into three steps, and all pain patients, regardless of the intensity of pain, start taking medication from the first step.

Based on patients' chief complaints and statements, combined with other medical history information, the degree of pain is objectively determined, and then a treatment plan is formulated. Auxiliary medications can be added if necessary, but the purpose of relieving pain must be achieved.

Misunderstanding 3: The intensity of pain should be determined by doctors, and patients' complaints should not be easily believed.

Pain is a subjective feeling that varies from person to person. Doctors must make standardized assessments, trust patients' feelings, and treat them accordingly.

Misunderstanding 4: All pain patients can only receive oral medications.

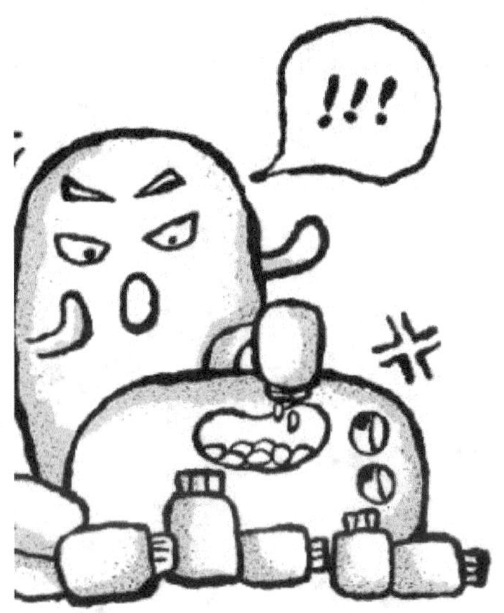

This is a misconception. With the development of medicine and the improvement of treatment level, in addition to oral administration, transdermal patches, mucosal agents, sublingual tablets, sprays, rectal suppositories and intravenous drips can be used. The specific choice should be based on the actual situation. Try to choose non-invasive routes, especially for patients who cannot take oral medication due to the disease itself, and should choose other methods.

Misunderstanding 5: It is enough to relieve the pain, there is no need to achieve pain-free.

Standardized pain management not only relieves pain, but also minimizes the adverse effects of drugs and improves the life quality of patients, allowing cancer patients to live a pain-free life (pain-free sleep, pain-free rest, and pain-free activities).

Misunderstanding 6: Cancer pain control is not important while tumor treatment is important.

Patients believe that cancer pain is normal and something they must endure. Once the tumor is cured, the pain will naturally go away. Analgesics are only used when the pain is severe. Long-term pain seriously affects the life quality of patients and their families.

Misunderstanding 7: Analgesic treatment is only given when there is pain.

Regardless of whether pain is present at the time of medication, using analgesics on time, maintaining effective blood drug concentrations, and improving the body's tolerance is not only safe and effective, but also requires the lowest intensity

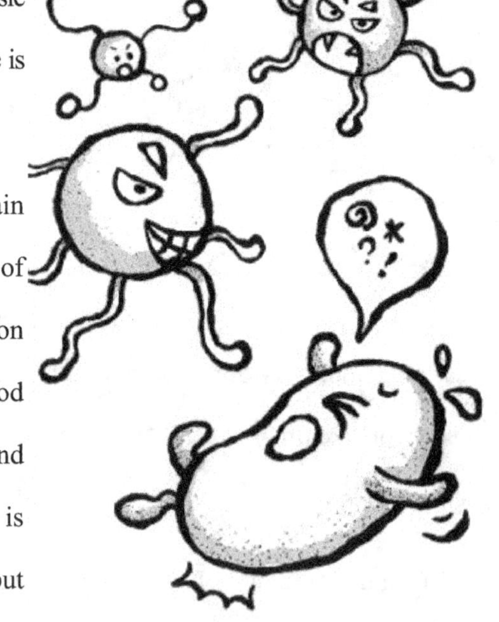

and dose of analgesics. On the contrary, cancer pain that has not received effective analgesic treatment for a long time is prone to sympathetic nerve dysfunction related to neuropathic pain caused by pain, manifested as refractory pain such as pain sensitivity and abnormal pain.

Misunderstanding 8: Opioids are highly toxic and non-opioid drugs are safer.

For patients who need long-term use of analgesics, opioids are safer and have no toxic effects on the liver, kidneys, heart, etc. In fact, except for the side effect of constipation, the adverse reactions of opioids are mostly temporary or tolerable.

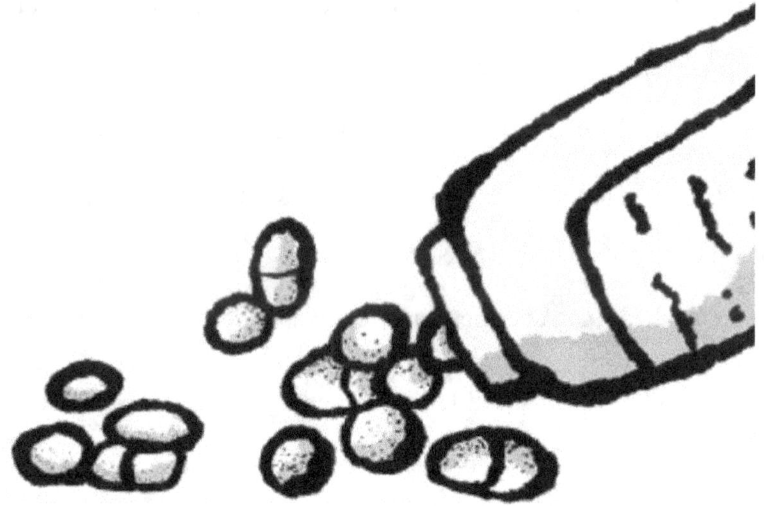

Misunderstanding 9: People with respiratory problems cannot take opioids.

Because the dyspnea caused by lung disease is caused by lung lesions, and opioids have a central effect on respiratory depression. Opioids themselves will not aggravate lung lesions. If opioids are used rationally, respiratory depression is rare.

Misunderstanding 10: Long-term use of opioid painkillers can cause addiction.

In fact, studies have shown that long-term use of opioid analgesics—especially timed oral administration—is less likely to lead to addiction. It is important to distinguish between true addiction and "pseudo addiction". Pseudo-addiction refers to a phenomenon in which patients exhibit drug-seeking behaviors due to inadequate pain relief from the prescribed dosage, also known as "iatrogenic syndrome." The root cause is insufficient analgesia. When the drug dose is increased and the pain is sufficiently relieved, drug-seeking behavior may disappear, and reasonable treatment can avoid it.

Incorrect concepts often lead to patients not following doctors' orders for medication, which is manifested by not using opioids as much as possible, using weak opioids instead, or reducing the dosage or frequency of use, etc., so that pain cannot be effectively controlled. As long as cancer patients strictly follow doctors' instructions and take controlled-release and sustained-release preparations of opioids for pain relief, they can ensure ideal analgesic treatment while keeping the incidence of addiction to less than 1%. Opioids, including morphine, are essential drugs for cancer pain treatment, and the "addictiveness" of such drugs is very rare.

Misunderstanding 11: If patients experience adverse reactions such as nausea, vomiting, and constipation after using opioids, patients should stop taking the drugs immediately.

In fact, nausea and vomiting usually only occur in the first few days of medication, and the symptoms usually disappear on their own after a few days; constipation can also be relieved through correct measures. There is no need to stop the medication when these adverse reactions occur, just actively prevent and treat them.

Misunderstanding 12: Pethidine is the best analgesic.

Dulantin, also known as pethidine hydrochloride. Many patients and family members believe that injecting Dulantin is the best way to relieve pain. In fact, the intensity of Dulantin's analgesic effect is only one-eighth to one-tenth that of morphine, and its duration of action is short. Long-term use of Dulantin for pain relief can easily lead to "addiction" in patients. Dulantin is listed as a drug that is not recommended for pain treatment. As early as 1996, the Ministry of Health of China explicitly stipulated that the use of Dulantin in cancer pain treatment is prohibited.

Part 9: Common Toxic and Side Effects of Chemotherapy and Simple Treatment and Care

The side effects of chemotherapy are categorized according to the system in which they occur, mainly into blood toxicity, gastrointestinal toxicity, lung toxicity, cardiotoxicity, liver toxicity, kidney toxicity, neurotoxicity, skin and appendage toxicity and others.

1. Bone marrow suppression

1. Drugs with significant bone marrow suppression

Taxanes (paclitaxel, docetaxel); vinca alkaloids (vindesine, vinorelbine); nitrosoureas (carmustine, cyclohexanenitrosourea, methylnitrosourea); anthracyclines (daunorubicin, doxorubicin).

2. Solutions

(1) Stop taking the medication.

(2) Prevent and treat infection.

(3) Orally take various drugs that help increase white blood cells, such as Leukojun tablets, leukoamine, shark liver alcohol, etc.

(4) The white blood cell count typically begins to decline approximately 1 week after drug discontinuation, reaches its nadir around day 10, and remains at a low level for 2–3 days before recovery begins. Normal levels are usually restored within 7–10 days. In general, Grade I–II leukopenia does not require intervention, as it typically resolves spontaneously and does not affect the next chemotherapy cycle. However, Grade III–IV leukopenia usually

necessitates active treatment. When the white blood cell count is severely reduced (above degree III), 200 µg of recombinant human granulocyte stimulating factor can be injected subcutaneously, 1 to 2 times a day, for 3 consecutive days.

(5) For patients with indications for blood transfusion, component blood transfusion should be given.

(6) Albumin and plasma infusion.

(7) Platelet counts decrease later than white blood cell counts but recover more rapidly. Currently, there are no highly effective pharmacological treatments for thrombocytopenia. Grade I and II platelet inhibition do not require treatment, while grade III and IV platelet inhibition requires active treatment. If platelets are significantly reduced in the short term, interleukin-11 can be injected subcutaneously and hemostatic drugs can be given to prevent bleeding.

2. Gastrointestinal symptoms

1. Drugs with obvious gastrointestinal reactions

Nausea and vomiting are more obvious after taking cisplatin, cyclophosphamide, etoposide, dacarbazine, and doxorubicin; diarrhea is often caused after taking fluorouracil, capecitabine, and irinotecan, and in severe cases, it can lead to death.

Vinca alkaloids (e.g., vincristine, vinblastine, and vinorelbine) often induce constipation. Notably, vincristine may occasionally lead to paralytic ileus.

2. Solutions

(1) Treatment of nausea and vomiting

The American Society of Clinical Oncology (ASCO) has updated its antiemetic regimen recommendations for the prevention and treatment of chemotherapy-induced nausea and vomiting.

To ensure the authoritativeness and clinical applicability of the guidelines, the expert panel was composed of oncologists, radiologists, nurses, pharmacists, health services researchers, and patient representatives. The panel conducted a systematic review of medical literature published between 2009 and 2016 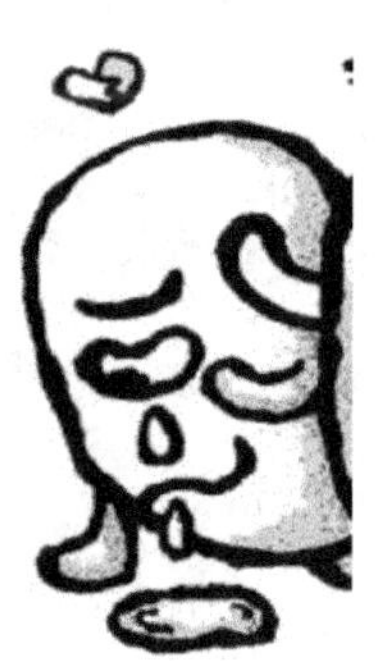 to develop evidence-based recommendations. Key recommendations include:

For adult patients at high risk of nausea and vomiting (e.g., those receiving cisplatin, cyclophosphamide, or anthracycline combinations), olanzapine should be added to the standard antiemetic regimen (typically a 5-HT3 receptor antagonist, NK1 receptor antagonist, and dexamethasone). Olanzapine may also be used prophylactically before chemotherapy.

For adults receiving carboplatin-based chemotherapy or high-dose chemotherapy, and for high-risk pediatric patients, an NK1 receptor antagonist should be incorporated into the standard regimen (5-HT3 receptor antagonist plus dexamethasone).

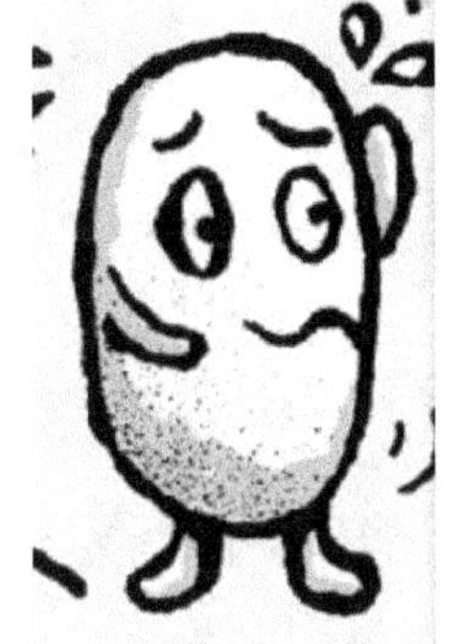

Additional guidance specifies:

Dexamethasone may be restricted to chemotherapy days for patients on anthracycline-cyclophosphamide regimens.

For refractory nausea/vomiting unresponsive to standard therapy, FDA-approved cannabinoids (dronabinol or nabilone) are recommended. However, insufficient evidence supports using medical marijuana for chemotherapy- or radiation-induced nausea/vomiting.

(2) Treatment of diarrhea

It is not common during chemotherapy, but some individual drugs can cause diarrhea: fluorouracil, capecitabine, and irinotecan.

Fluorouracil-induced diarrhea occurs due to its suppression of Escherichia coli (the predominant intestinal bacteria), which subsequently promotes the overgrowth of drug-resistant organisms - most notably Clostridium difficile. Live bacterial preparations can be given to increase the number of negative bacilli in the intestine. When pseudomembranous colitis is highly suspected, antidiarrheal drugs must not be given, as this will aggravate the symptoms of intestinal poisoning. In this case, medication should be taken in a timely manner according to doctors' advice.

(3) Constipation

Vinca alkaloids such as vincristine, vinblastine amide, and vinblastine can cause constipation. Patients can eat more fiber-rich foods, fresh fruits and vegetables, and use laxatives when necessary.

(4) Loss of appetite

It is the initial reaction to chemotherapy drugs and occurs 1 to 2 days after chemotherapy. Generally, no special treatment is required. Progesterone drugs can relieve symptoms.

3. Hepatotoxicity

1. Drugs that can cause hepatotoxicity

Nitrosourea drugs, 6-mercaptopurine, cytarabine, asparaginase, and dacarbazine can all cause hepatotoxicity.

2. Solutions

(1) Acute mild hepatotoxicity typically develops 1-2 weeks post-chemotherapy and is generally self-limiting. Clinical manifestations include elevated liver transaminases and bilirubin, with occasional jaundice. Treatment mainly includes: stopping chemotherapy or postponing chemotherapy (generally resumes after 1 week); giving liver-protecting drugs; giving enzyme-lowering drugs; and giving polarizing fluids (which are beneficial for jaundice). Recheck liver enzyme levels one week after

treatment, and chemotherapy can be resumed if they are normal.

(2) Use of liver protection drugs:

(i) Reduced glutathione

Dissolve 1.5 g/m^2 reduced glutathione in 100 mL of 0.9% sodium chloride solution within 15 minutes before chemotherapy, and infuse intravenously within 15 minutes. In the second to fifth days, inject 600 mg intramuscularly every day. When using cyclophosphamide (CTX), in order to prevent damage to the urinary system, it is recommended to complete the infusion within 15 minutes immediately after the injection of CTX.

(ii) Polyene phosphatidylcholine

Generally infuse 10 mg per day while for severe cases, the dosage can be increased to 20mg per day; dilution with electrolyte solutions (0.9% sodium chloride solution, Ringer's solution, etc.) is strictly prohibited; if intravenous infusion is to be prepared, it can only be diluted with glucose solution without electrolytes (such as 5%/10% glucose solution, 5% xylitol solution); if other infusions are to be prepared, the pH value of the mixed solution must not be lower than 7.5, and the prepared solution must remain clear during the infusion process.

4. Nephrotoxicity

1. Drugs that cause nephrotoxicity

Common drugs that cause kidney and bladder toxicity include cisplatin, cyclophosphamide, ifosfamide, methotrexate, and mitomycin.

Cisplatin: It has the greatest impact on the kidneys, mainly causing damage to the renal tubules, which is irreversible in a sense. Endless use of cisplatin chemotherapy will lead to glomerular damage and eventually renal failure.

Ifosfamide: Hemorrhagic cystitis is the most serious side effect caused by it and is an indication for stopping chemotherapy.

2. Solutions

Preventive measures for chemotherapy-induced nephrotoxicity include: (1) regular renal function monitoring and maintenance of adequate hydration; (2) using combination chemotherapy to minimize individual drug doses; (3) avoiding aminoglycoside antibiotics during cisplatin treatment. For high-dose cisplatin, implement hydration and diuresis protocols, and consider the cell membrane protector amifostine to mitigate toxicity. Methotrexate requires special precautions due to direct renal toxicity - after high-dose administration, monitor blood drug concentrations and implement calcium folinate rescue therapy with hydration and urine alkalinization. For ifosfamide and high-dose cyclophosphamide, their metabolite acrolein can cause hemorrhagic cystitis; this can be prevented by prophylactic administration of sodium 2-mercaptoethanesulfonate (mesna).

5. Cardiotoxicity

1. Drugs that cause cardiotoxicity

Anthracyclines (doxorubicin, epirubicin) have an effect on the myocardium, and this effect will not disappear for a long time. Paclitaxel has an effect on the conduction system of the heart. High-dose cyclophosphamide can cause myocarditis, and the toxicity is aggravated when combined with anthracyclines.

2. Solutions

Many anti-tumor drugs have certain toxic effects on the heart, mainly anthracycline antibiotics, among which doxorubicin is the most important, which can cause a dose-related cardiomyopathy. If these drugs are used, ECG monitoring must be performed and heart function should be tested regularly.

Among the factors that affect the cardiotoxicity of doxorubicin, the cumulative total dose is the most important risk factor. Liposomal doxorubicin has low cardiotoxicity and is a good choice.

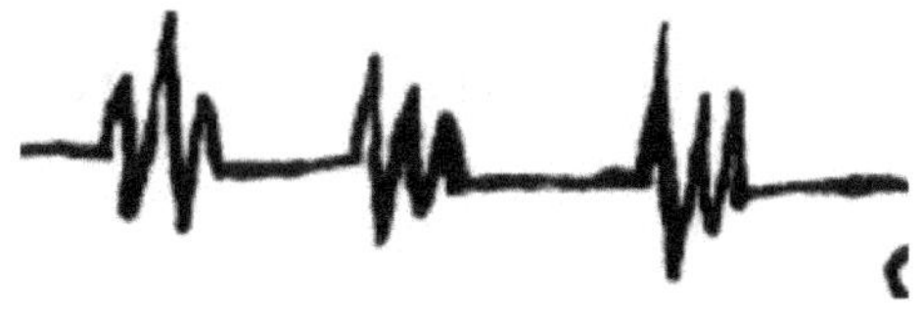

Anthracycline-induced cardiomyopathy can be clinically divided into two types:

(1) Acute myopericarditis: usually occurs within a few days of medication, manifested as transient arrhythmia, pericardial effusion and myocardial dysfunction. Occasionally, it may lead to transient heart failure and death.

(2) Subacute cardiac toxicity: The onset is insidious, and symptoms may appear after the last dose of the drug, but the most common onset is 3 months after the last dose. Clinical manifestations may include tachycardia and fatigue, and finally emphysema, right heart congestion, and decreased cardiac output. The use of cardiotonic drugs can stabilize the condition. Treatment of anthracycline-induced cardiomyopathy usually requires intravenous medication to enhance myocardial contractility and reduce the afterload of the heart. Angiotensin-converting enzyme inhibitors play an important role in stabilizing heart failure and delaying the deterioration of cardiomyopathy. Selective beta-blockers can also be used for those who are ineffective.

The manifestations of cardiotoxicity of continuous infusion of high-dose fluorouracil may include: precordial pain, ST-T changes, atrial arrhythmias, myocardial infarction, heart failure, and sudden death. The effects of DDP on the heart may include atrial fibrillation, angina pectoris, and ST-T changes.

Prevention is the key clinical approach for chemotherapy-induced heart disease. Doctors often add cardioprotectants when using cardiotoxic chemotherapy drugs.

6. Pulmonary toxicity

1. Drugs that cause lung toxicity

Drugs that are likely to cause pulmonary fibrosis include: bleomycin, bleomycin, high-dose carmustine, high-dose cyclophosphamide, gemcitabine, etc.

2. Solutions

Patients of advanced age, those with poor lung function, or chronic bronchitis should exercise caution or avoid using drugs with a high risk of pulmonary toxicity. The dosage of related drugs should be strictly controlled: (i) bleomycin (BLM) should not exceed 300 mg; (ii) carmustine (BCNU) should not exceed 1500 mg/m^2; (iii) lomustine (CCNU) should not exceed 1100 mg/m^2. Steroid corticosteroid treatment may be effective.

7. Neurotoxicity

1. Drugs that cause neurotoxicity

(1) Peripheral neuritis

(i) Peripheral nerves: oxaliplatin, vinca alkaloids, taxanes, etoposide and teniposide.

(ii) Central nervous system: Ifosfamide and fluorouracil may cause cerebellar ataxia.

(2) Auditory nerve damage

Cisplatin is the chemotherapy drug most likely to cause auditory nerve damage. If such toxicity occurs, discontinuation of cisplatin is recommended.

2. Solutions

Peripheral neurotoxicity is often reversible. For severe cases, the drug should be discontinued in time. High-dose vitamin supplementation may alleviate the symptoms. Giving B vitamins during chemotherapy breaks is beneficial to alleviate peripheral nerve symptoms.

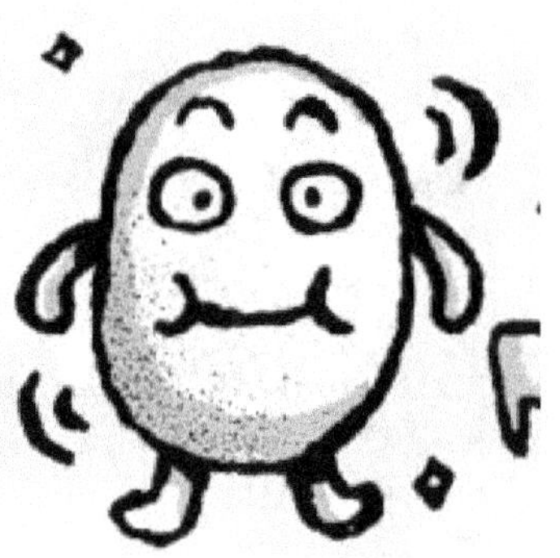

Severe peripheral neuritis is an indication for stopping chemotherapy. If patients complain of auditory nerve damage, an otolaryngologist should be consulted immediately and a hearing test should be performed if necessary. As a general rule, furosemide should be avoided during cisplatin chemotherapy, as it may potentiate cisplatin-induced ototoxicity.

8. Skin toxicity

1. Drugs that cause skin toxicity

(1) Allergic reaction

Many chemotherapy drugs can cause allergic reactions, with common drugs including bleomycin, doxorubicin, and cisplatin. Once it occurs, the drug should be stopped immediately. Some chemotherapy drugs, such as paclitaxel drugs, must be treated accordingly before use. They are transient erythema and urticaria, which often appear within a few hours after taking the drug, last for a few hours and disappear, and sometimes occur a few days after taking the drug.

(2) Stomatitis

Common drugs associated with stomatitis include methotrexate, fluorouracil, cyclophosphamide, mitomycin, dacarbazine, doxorubicin, vinblastine, and vincristine. Among which methotrexate and fluorouracil are the most common.

(3) Skin pigmentation

It is often confined to the nail bed, oral mucosa or the area of medicated veins. Common drugs include doxorubicin, bleomycin, fluorouracil, cyclophosphamide, carmustine, daunorubicin, etc.

(4) Skin keratosis

Long-term bleomycin use may lead to skin thickening, particularly on the palms, soles, face, and areas of trauma. In severe cases, this can impair hand function. Fluorouracil can sometimes cause hand-foot syndrome, which is characterized by erythematous peeling of the palms and soles, often accompanied by pain.

2. Solutions

Oral ulcers are a manifestation of digestive tract ulcers, indicating that other parts of the digestive tract have also been ulcerated. They begin to appear 5 to 6 days after taking the medicine and gradually heal after about a week of stopping the medicine. Ulcers caused by anti-metabolites are mostly found on the lip and cheek mucosa. For severe cases, they can extend to the pharynx, esophagus and even the anus, and a few can affect the vaginal opening and urethra. Ulcers caused by dactinomycin are mostly on the sides and roots of the tongue, with deep ulcers and severe pain.

For oral care, irrigate ulcerated areas with high-pressure 0.9% sodium chloride solution to remove surface secretions and necrotic tissue before applying topical medication. Encourage speech as it promotes ulcer healing. Monitor body temperature closely and watch for worsening local infections, which may progress to systemic infection. Administer antibiotics promptly when indicated, including specific coverage for anaerobic organisms when necessary.

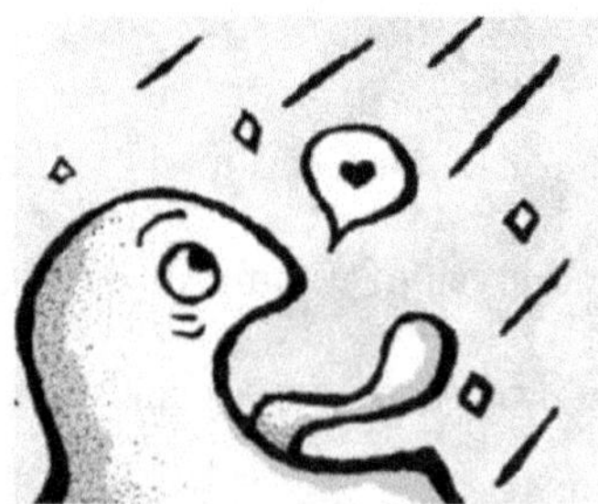

The primary objectives in managing stomatitis are pain relief and infection prevention. Initial management should focus on maintaining oral hygiene. For pain control, systemic analgesics may be administered, or topical anesthetics such as procaine, lidocaine, or Bingpeng Powder can be applied. In cases of secondary infection, appropriate antibiotic therapy (either systemic or topical) should be initiated.

Take 0.2% chlorhexidine or dexamethasone 10 mg, gentamicin 160,000U 0.9% sodium chloride solution for gargling before eating, 10-15 mL each time, 0.5-1 minute. If fungal infection is suspected, gargle with 5% sodium bicarbonate or nystatin, and anaerobic bacteria with hydrogen peroxide.

Mild skin keratosis does not affect chemotherapy and can be recovered after stopping treatment, but for severe skin keratosis, drug administration must be stopped.

9. Hair loss

1. Drugs that cause hair loss

The drugs most likely to cause hair loss are antibiotic chemotherapy drugs, such as dactinomycin, doxorubicin, epirubicin, bleomycin, and bleomycin. In addition, antimetabolites and plant alkaloid chemotherapy

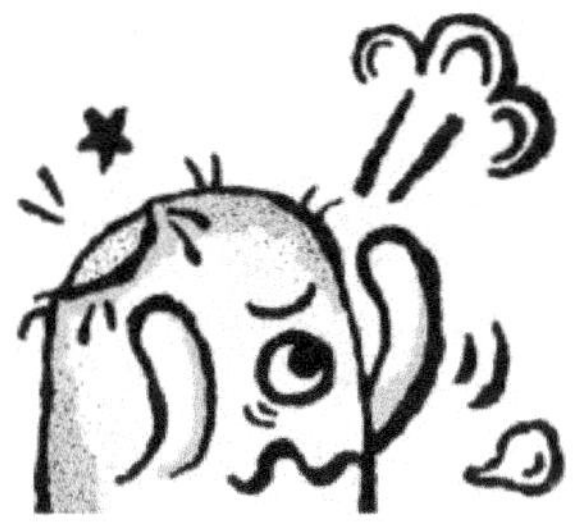

solutions are prone to hair loss, such as Taxol, VP-16, and VCR.

2. Solutions

Hair loss is the most common side effect of chemotherapy. It typically begins 1-2 weeks after treatment initiation, peaks around 2 months, and starts to regrow within 1-2 months after chemotherapy completion. To minimize discomfort, patients should: Avoid irritating shampoos; avoid hair dryers, curling irons, hair spray, hair dyes, and excessive hair combing; clean up hair loss on the bed in time; patients can use wigs to relieve negative emotions; more important for patients is psychological treatment, so that patients understand that they will grow very good hair after chemotherapy stops, and the hair quality will not be worse than before.

10. Local irritation

1. Drugs that cause local irritation

Various plant-based chemotherapy drugs: such as vincristine, etoposide, paclitaxel, topotecan; antibiotic chemotherapy drugs: doxorubicin, epirubicin, bleomycin, dactinomycin; antimetabolites: fluorouracil, methotrexate; the drugs most likely to cause skin damage are anthracyclines (doxorubicin, epirubicin), which are of course the most serious.

2. Solutions

Once drug extravasation occurs, local blockade (procaine+0.9% sodium chloride solution/procaine+0.9% chlorine solution+ dexamethasone/ice pack for local cold compress) is performed.

Part 10: Chemotherapy Emergencies and Nursing

1. Chemotherapy extravasation

Chemotherapy drugs are highly toxic and irritating, and extravasation of the drugs can often cause serious consequences. What should we do if it happens?

1. Treatment of drug extravasation

Extravasation of chemotherapy drugs can cause local pain, local tissue swelling, ulceration and necrosis, or the formation of local nodules.

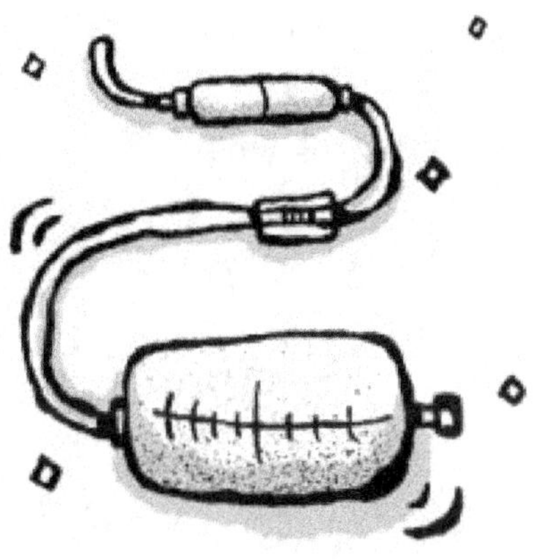

The general principles for the treatment of extravasation of intravenous drugs are: (i) stop the infusion; (ii)raise the limb; (iii)keep the needle and withdraw the extravasated drug; (iv) inject 5-10 mL of 0.9% sodium chloride solution to dilute the exuded drug; (v) apply antidote locally; (vi) apply topical steroid hormones; (vii) 2% procaine local seal; (viii) cold compress; (ix) apply local Chinese medicine Glauber's salt powder or magnesium sulfate, or apply thin potato slices or cucumber slices.

2. Treatment of phlebitis

Phlebitis typically manifests initially with medication extravasation, progressing to venous induration and cord-like induration accompanied by localized cutaneous hyperpigmentation. In severe cases, affected extremities may develop paresthesia, edema, and pain. Preventive measures include: (i) Utilizing high-grade intravenous access (preferably central venous catheters) for chemotherapy administration; (ii) Ensuring proper drug reconstitution to recommended concentrations; (iii) Meticulously controlling infusion rates. For treatment, local hot compresses combined with topical Hirudoid cream application can help alleviate symptoms and promote recovery.

2. Allergic reactions

Allergic reactions to paclitaxel occur frequently, with an incidence of 10% to 20%. The key is to take preventive measures and keep anti-allergic drugs ready at all times. Routine pretreatment with corticosteroid dexamethasone tablets and antihistamine diphenhydramine before medication can reduce or prevent allergic reactions. Additionally, other chemotherapy agents may also cause hypersensitivity reactions.

In acute allergic reactions, management should not await laboratory confirmation. Epinephrine, oxygen therapy, nebulizer inhalation, β^2 receptor agonists, antihistamines and other treatments should be given as soon as possible.

1. Adrenaline first

Patients with laryngeal edema, bronchospasm, and urticaria should be given an immediate intramuscular injection of 0.3-0.5 mL of 1: 1000 epinephrine dilution, and repeated every 10-15 minutes if necessary, for a total of 3 times. If patients have severe hypotension, severe bronchospasm, severe upper respiratory tract edema and other critical conditions, a one-time intravenous injection of 0.5-1.0 mL of 1:10000 epinephrine dilution can be given (the dose can be repeated after an interval of 10-15 minutes).

After the above treatment, if the symptoms are still not significantly improved, epinephrine can be continuously infused intravenously at a rate of 1-4 Pg/min until patients' symptoms are relieved. If intravenous access cannot be established within a short period of time, intratracheal administration can be performed in an emergency, and the dose is twice the above intravenous dose.

2. Oxygen therapy

If patients have difficulty breathing, he/she can be given oxygen by mask. Intubation can be given when severe drowsiness and hypoxemia occur. If patients have upper airway edema and cannot be intubated, a tracheotomy is required. The target value of oxygen therapy is blood oxygen saturation > 90% (PaO^2 > 60 mmHg).

3. Bronchodilators

For patients with persistent bronchospasm, nebulized albuterol may be used.

4. Antihistamines

After epinephrine treatment, diphenhydramine 25 to 50 mg IV, IM, or orally every 4 to 6 hours and cimetidine 50 mg IV or 150 mg orally every 8 hours (or other H^2 receptor antagonists) may be given to help reduce the release of histamine and further relieve hypotension and mild urticaria-related symptoms.

5. Glucocorticoids

Patients who have bronchospasm due to an allergic reaction may be treated with glucocorticoids. The first dose is methylprednisolone 120 mg IV once, followed by 60 mg IV every 6 hours. These hormone treatments also help reduce the late symptoms of an allergic reaction (which may appear 6 to 12 hours after the early symptoms).

6. Circulation support

Hypotension typically responds to epinephrine treatment. However, for patients whose blood pressure does not improve after epinephrine administration, intravenous 0.9% sodium chloride (normal saline) solution may be given for volume expansion. For patients who still have refractory hypotension after active volume supplementation, vasopressors such as norepinephrine or epinephrine can be given to maintain it if necessary.

7. ECG monitoring

Patients who require epinephrine treatment for an allergic reaction should be closely monitored and may need admission to an intensive care unit (ICU) for observation. Sometimes the disease recurs and may not appear until several hours after the early symptoms appear, so monitoring should be continued for at least 24 hours before it can be withdrawn.

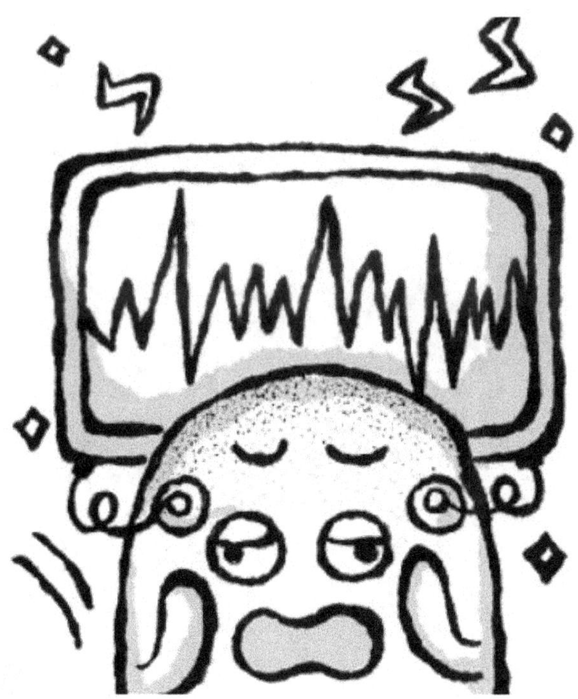

Part 11: Daily Care of Central Venous Catheters

Intravenous therapy is a medical treatment method that involves injecting various drugs (including blood products) and blood into the blood circulation through the veins. It includes intravenous injection, intravenous infusion and intravenous blood transfusion. Commonly used tools include: syringes, infusion (blood) devices, disposable intravenous infusion needles, peripheral venous indwelling needles, central venous catheters, peripherally inserted central venous catheters, infusion ports and infusion assist devices, etc.

1. Common central venous catheters

1. Central venous catheter (CVC)

A central venous catheter (CVC) is inserted through the subclavian vein, internal jugular vein, or femoral vein, with its tip positioned in the superior vena cava (SVC) or inferior vena cava (IVC).

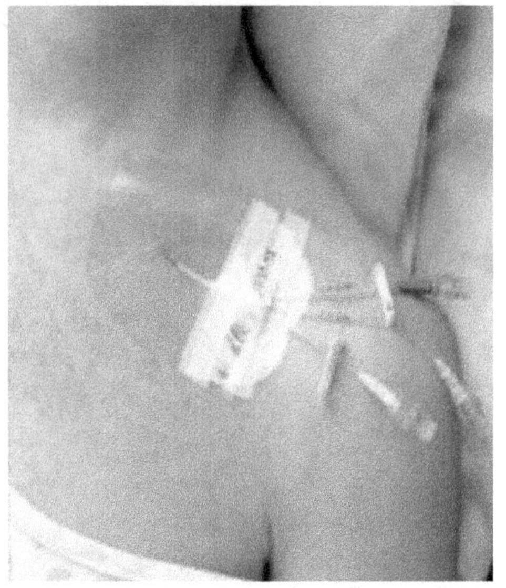

CVC

2. Peripherally inserted central catheter (PICC)

The catheter is inserted

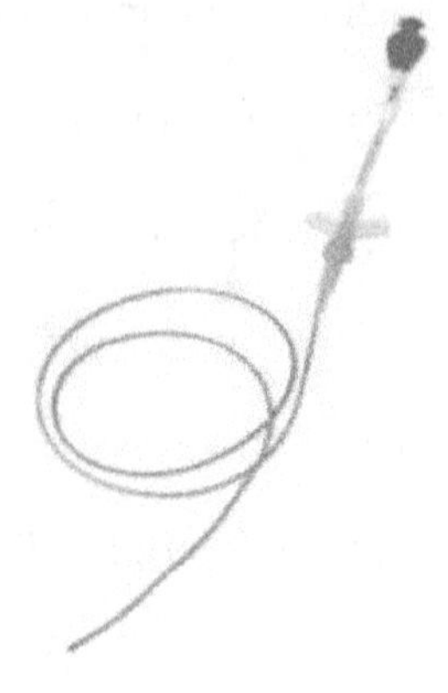

through puncture into the veins of the upper limb, median cubital vein, cephalic vein, brachial vein, and external jugular vein (for newborns, it can also be inserted through the great saphenous vein of the lower limb, temporal vein of the head, posterior auricular vein, etc.), with the tip of the catheter located in the superior vena cava or inferior vena cava.

3. Port

A fully implantable closed infusion system consists of: (i) A catheter with its tip positioned in the superior vena cava (SVC), and (ii) A subcutaneously implanted injection port. This device is a totally implantable venous access system comprising a central venous catheter (terminating in the SVC) and a subcutaneous infusion port.

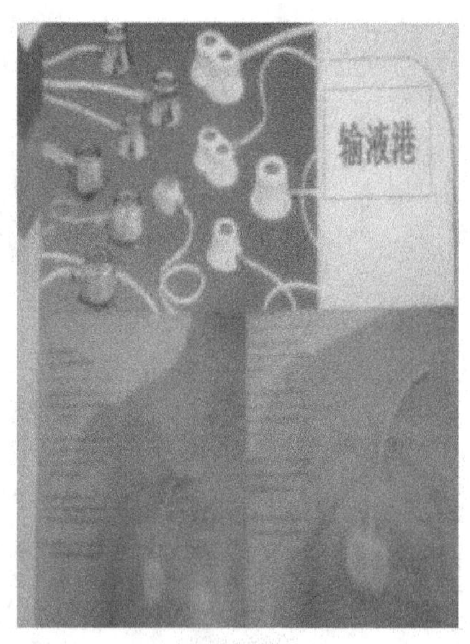

PORT

2. Management of complications related to intravenous therapy

1. Phlebitis

(1) The PICC can be retained temporarily; go to the hospital promptly and receive symptomatic treatment as prescribed by doctors.

(2) Raise and immobilize the affected limb to avoid pressure. If necessary, stop intravenous infusion in the affected limb.

(3) Changes in local and systemic conditions should be observed and recorded.

2. Drug exudation and drug extravasation

(1) Immediately stop infusion at the original site, elevate the affected limb, notify medical staff promptly, and provide symptomatic treatment.

(2) Observe and record changes in skin color, temperature, sensation, joint movement, and distal blood circulation in the area of exudation or extravasation.

3. Catheter-related venous thrombosis

(1) If catheter-related venous thrombosis is suspected, elevate and immobilize the affected limb. Avoid heat application, massage, or compression. Seek immediate medical evaluation and follow the physician's instructions for symptomatic treatment, ensuring proper documentation of the condition.

(2) The swelling, pain, skin temperature and color, bleeding tendency and functional activities of the limb, shoulder, neck and chest on the side where the catheter is placed should be observed.

4. Catheter blockage

(1) When the intravenous catheter is blocked, the cause of the blockage should be analyzed and 0.9% sodium chloride solution should not be forcefully injected.

(2) When catheter blockage is confirmed, PICC, CVC, and PORT should be handled and recorded in a timely manner.

5. Catheter-related bloodstream infection

If a catheter-related bloodstream infection is suspected, immediately discontinue the infusion, leave the PICC/CVC/PORT catheter in place temporarily, and follow the physician's orders to obtain blood cultures and initiate appropriate treatment.

6. Infusion reaction

(1) When an infusion reaction occurs, the infusion should be stopped, the drug solution and infusion set should be replaced, symptomatic treatment should be given, and the original drug solution and infusion set should be retained.

(2) Changes in patients' condition should be closely observed and

recorded.

7. Exudate from the puncture site

(1) Care should be taken to protect the skin around the puncture site.

(2) Local pressure can be applied to the puncture site to reduce the amount of exudate.

(3) Temporarily retain the PICC, CVC, and PORT and notify doctors to provide symptomatic treatment.

8. Catheter pressure injury

(1) Care should be taken to protect the skin around the puncture site.

(2) A high-lift platform method or sterile pad can be used to assist in fixing the vascular access device (VAD).

3. What should patients with indwelling central venous catheters pay attention to?

1. Pay attention to PICC placement

(1) Self-care after PICC placement

(i) Keep the area clean and dry, and do not remove the film without authorization.

(ii) Please promptly contact your doctor if any of the following occur after catheterization: the film becomes curled, loose, or damp; the puncture site and surrounding area become red, swollen, painful, or exudates; the PICC leakage scale changes; rash, blisters, or itching on the skin around the puncture site; pain or swelling in the punctured upper limb, etc.

(iii) During infusion, the limb on the side with the catheter should be placed freely and appropriately elevated. When sleeping, maintain a comfortable position and try to avoid compressing the limb on the side with the catheter.

(iv) Before showering, use a PICC protective cover or plastic wrap to tightly wrap the film 10 cm above and below, and avoid soaking the film.

(v) During the treatment interval or after discharge, go to the hospital every 5 to 7 days to replace the film and exposed connector and flush the tube to maintain the PICC functional status.

(2) Functional training after PICC placement

(i) Clean the elastic bandage and loosen it after 2 hours. If there is any swelling or discomfort, please contact the nurse at any time.

(ii) Gently move the wrist and elbow joints of the upper limb on the catheter-placed side every day. It is advised to make a fist, rotate the wrist, and raise and abduct the upper limb. Avoid excessive force and insist on taking a walk indoors and outdoors every day.

(iii) The limb on the side with the catheter can carry out daily activities, but does not lift heavy objects or participate in strenuous sports such as playing badminton.

(iv) It is recommended to drink more than 1000 mL of water every day, and soak hands and feet in warm water every morning and evening. Use comfortably warm water to avoid thermal injury. Bedridden patients should maintain adequate activity and can accept passive exercises such as massage.

2. Pay attention to the indwelling CVC

(1) During the catheterization period, patients should avoid showering to prevent water from penetrating the dressing and causing infection.

(2) While the catheter is in place, the neck can be moved normally, such as turning left and right, and nodding up and down. Do not bend the neck excessively to prevent the tube from being bent and affecting the smooth infusion of the fluid.

(3) When patients turn over and move, pay attention to protect the catheter to prevent it from slipping out; if the catheter accidentally slips out, immediately press the puncture point, do not move at will, and notify the medical staff immediately.

(4) If experiencing pain, itching, or other discomfort at the puncture site, medical staff should be contacted promptly.

(5) If the dressing is damp, contaminated, bleeding, exuding, damaged in integrity or peeled off, it should be replaced by medical staff in a timely manner.

(6) The infusion drip rate cannot be adjusted at will.

3. Pay attention to the port

(1) Purple spots may appear at the site of catheter placement and disappear on their own in 1 to 2 weeks.

(2) After the wound has healed, patients can take a bath and continue their daily life as usual, but avoid strenuous movement of the limb on the puncture side and avoid hitting the puncture site.

(3) After discharge, patients with PORT should go to the hospital every 4 weeks to receive catheter flushing with heparin diluent to avoid catheter blockage. It is recommended to review chest X-ray every 3 to 6 months.

(4) If the skin at the PORT becomes red, swollen, hot, or painful, it indicates subcutaneous infection or leakage and patients must return to the hospital for treatment. Edema and pain in the shoulder, neck, and ipsilateral upper limb should be checked promptly.

(5) Do not flush the catheter with force and avoid high-pressure injection.

(6) When using and maintaining the instrument, a syringe with a capacity of 10 mL or more must be used.

(7) The infusion pump pressure should not exceed 25 Pa during infusion.

(8) The patch applied after needle removal should be kept for 24 to 72

hours before being removed, and bathing can be done 72 hours after needle removal.

Part 12: What is Radiotherapy?

1.   What is radiotherapy?

Radiotherapy is a localized cancer treatment that utilizes radiation to target tumors. The accumulation of doses causes a series of chemical, physical, and biological changes within tumor tissue, leading to tumor shrinkage or even disappearance.

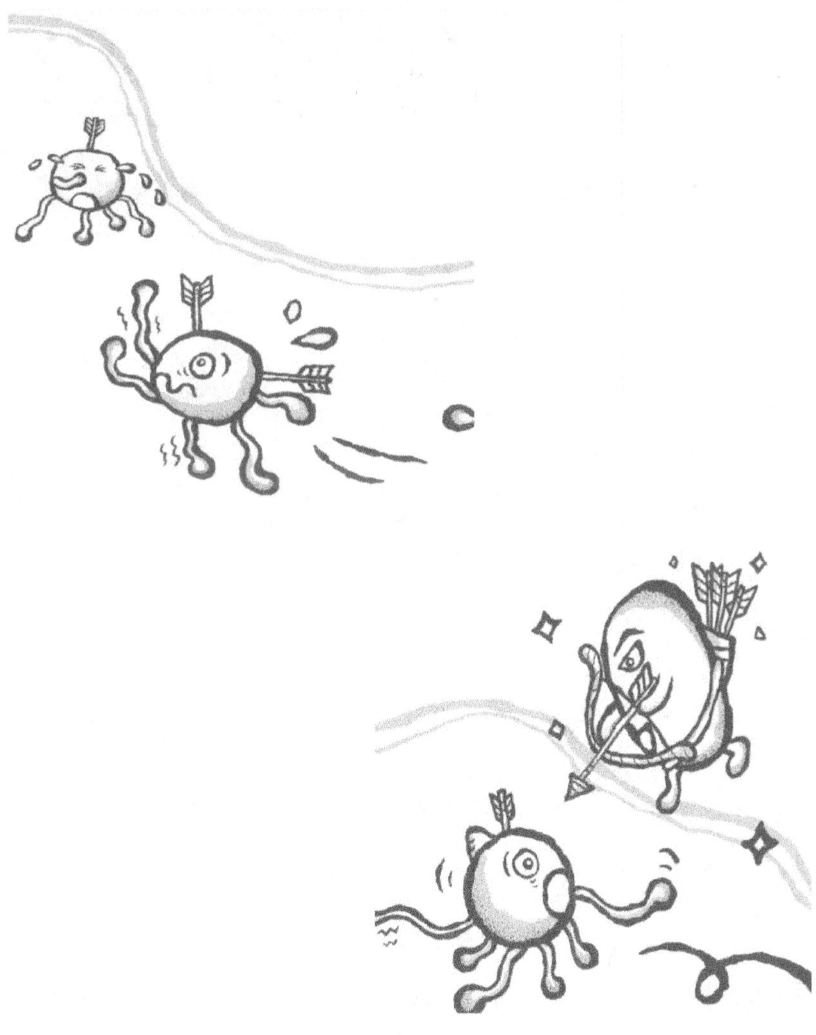

2.   Objectives of radiotherapy

The aim of radiotherapy is to effectively kill tumor cells while minimizing damage to surrounding healthy tissues. (Figure 1: Schematic diagram of radiotherapy).

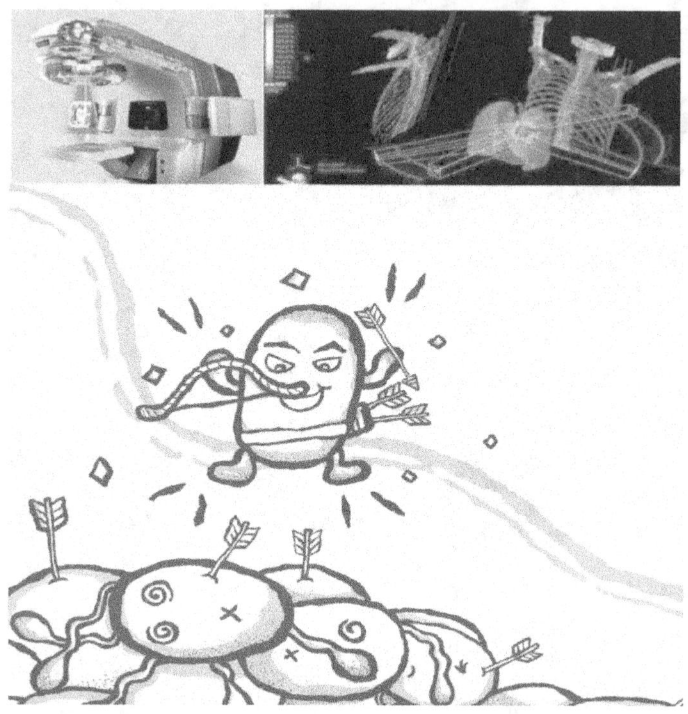

3. Common radiotherapy equipment

Low-energy X-ray superficial radiotherapy machines, cobalt-60 radiotherapy machines, conventional high-energy linear accelerators, precision-focused conformal radiotherapy equipment, after-loading brachytherapy devices and advanced proton and heavy ion radiotherapy equipment, etc.

4. Radiaotherapy Indications

(I) Based on tumor radiosensitivity

1. Highly radiosensitive tumors

Malignant lymphoma, testicular seminoma, Wilms tumor, neuroblastoma, medulloblastoma, Ewing sarcoma, small cell lung cancer, etc.

2. Moderately radiosensitive tumors

Head and neck squamous cell carcinoma, esophageal squamous cell carcinoma, lung squamous cell carcinoma, cervical cancer, endometrial cancer, breast cancer, skin cancer, renal transitional cell carcinoma, etc.

3. Tumors with low radiosensitivity

Gastrointestinal adenocarcinoma, pancreatic cancer, prostate cancer, etc.

4. Tumors with poor radiosensitivity

Most tumors originating from mesenchymal tissue, such as fibrosarcoma, liposarcoma, rhabdomyosarcoma, and malignant fibrous histiocytoma, etc.

(II) Organ-preserving radiotherapy.

Radiotherapy can achieve radical curative effects while preserving organ structure and function. For example, in breast-conserving surgery for early breast cancer, radical radiotherapy is required post-surgery, which not only achieves the same curative effect as radical surgery while preserving the breasts' structure and functions, with superior cosmetic outcomes. This type of tumor also includes: early-stage laryngeal cancer, low rectal cancer following sphincter-preserving surgery, and extremity soft tissue tumors.

(III) Combined radiotherapy and surgery

Preoperative radiotherapy can reduce tumor stage and improve surgical resection rates, for conditions such as breast cancer, rectal cancer, head and neck cancer and tumors with positive postoperative margins in various parts.

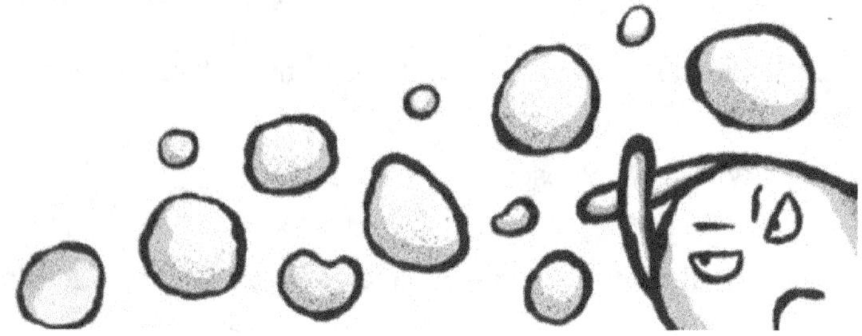

(IV) Palliative radiotherapy

For advanced tumors with distant metastasis to the bone or brain, or local tumor recurrence, radiotherapy is the most important palliative treatment. It can reduce pain, alleviate symptoms and improve quality of life without significant added toxicity. Following treatment, many patients can live with the tumor for several years or longer.

(V) Radiotherapy for benign conditions

Radiotherapy (alone or combined with surgery) yields favorable outcomes for select benign lesions such as hemangiomas and keloids.

5. Contraindications for radiotherapy

Radiotherapy has a few absolute contraindications. However, strict pre-treatment evaluation remains essential to avoid unnecessary physical and psychological burdens on patients. Radiotherapy is generally contraindicated under the following circumstances:

(I) General patient condition

1. Severe impairment of vital organ function, such as heart, liver, and kidneys, etc.

2. Uncontrolled systemic infections, septicemia or sepsis;

3. Uncorrected pre-treatment anemia (hemoglobin <80 g/L) or leukopenia (white blood cell count $<3.0\times10^9$/L)

4. Advanced cancer complicated with anemia, emaciation or cachexia where the predicted survival is < 3-6 months;

(II) Tumor characteristics

1. Widely metastatic advanced tumors with poor radiosensitivity, whose symptoms cannot be alleviated by radiotherapy;

2. Tumors with risk of visceral perforation or established perforation;

3. Radioresistant tumors, generally considered relative contraindications.

(III) Radiotherapy history/status

1. Recent history of radiotherapy;

2. Cutaneous or local tissue fibrosis;

3. Non-malignant skin ulcers confirmed by pathology;

4. Cases where additional radiotherapy is medically inadvisable.

Part 13: Preparing for Radiotherapy

1. Radiotherapy guidelines

(1) Adhere strictly to your radiation oncologist's treatment schedule. Do not arbitrarily modify the number of radiation sessions.

(2) Patients are not allowed to bring any metal objects when entering the radiotherapy room. Please remove all of them before entering, including phones, watches, pens, and jewelry. Patients with metal dentures must remove them.

(3) Maintain the positioning established by your radiation therapist throughout treatment. Do not move at will until the session concludes to ensure targeting accuracy.

(4) Keep radiation field marks clearly visible. If markings are unclear or blurred, request re-marking by your radiation oncologist before continuing treatment.

(5) Keep the irradiated skin clean. Wear soft cotton clothing, avoid soap, alcohol-based products, or scratching; gently pat dry sweat with a soft towel—do not rub; do not peel flaking skin or apply adhesive tapes.

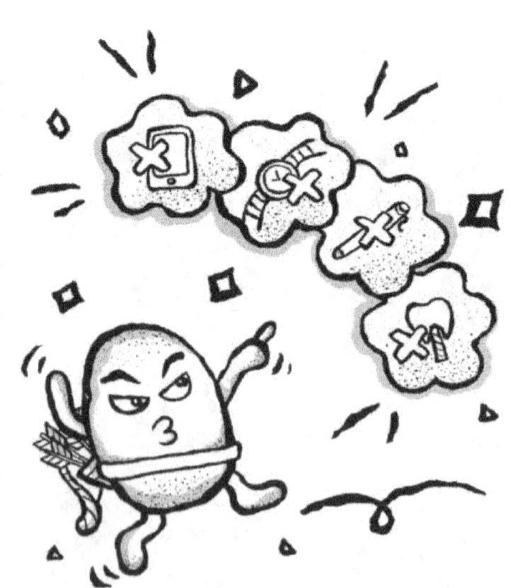

(6) Protect irradiated skin.

Avoid direct sunlight and stimulation such as overheating or overcooling. Do not apply irritants, such as alcohol and iodine, etc.

(7) Strengthen nutrition. Consume easily digestible foods, supplement a large amount of vitamins, eat more fresh vegetables and fruits, avoid spicy foods and strictly abstain from alcohol and tobacco.

(8) In order to excrete harmful substances released by the rupture and death of a large number of tumor cells caused by radiotherapy and reduce the reaction of systemic radiotherapy, patients should drink more water after radiotherapy, more than 3000 mL per day, to increase urine output. If necessary, give intravenous fluid replacement according to doctors' advice.

(9) During radiotherapy, you may experience systemic and/or local

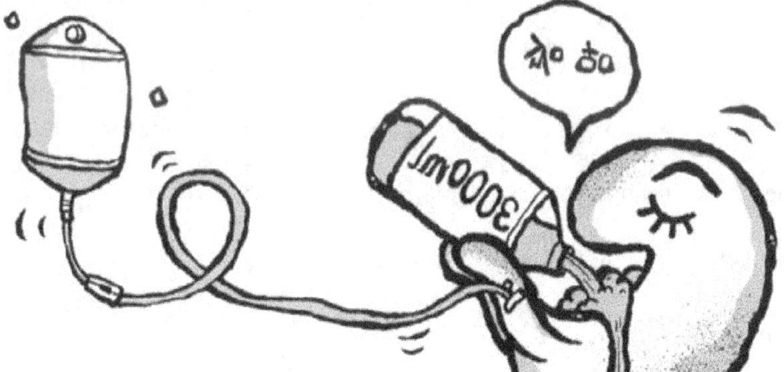

reactions. Common side effects include decreased white blood cells and thrombocytopenia. Blood tests should be checked 1 to 2 times weekly. If results fall below normal levels, suspend treatment as advised by your radiation oncologist. Take precautions to prevent colds and infections.

2. Radiotherapy preparation

(I) Pre-radiotherapy

1. Physical preparation guidance

Have your hair cut, beard shaved, nails trimmed, and skin cleansed through bathing before radiotherapy. Avoid skin scratches. During radiotherapy, do not wear metal-decorated clothing or metal accessories. Patients with metal tracheal tubes should switch to plastic or silicone tubes. Head radiotherapy patients must remove metal dental braces beforehand. Inform your doctor if metal stents are implanted. Metal objects generate secondary electrons during radiotherapy, increasing radiation dose to adjacent tissues and causing difficult-to-heal ulcers.

2. General preparation

Patients in poor general condition (e.g., anemia, infection, electrolyte imbalance, dehydration, myelosuppression) should receive symptomatic treatment before radiotherapy initiation.

(II) During radiotherapy

1. Radiation field skin protection

Wear soft, loose-fitting, moisture-absorbent cotton undergarments throughout treatment, avoid skin friction and maintain skin dryness/cleanliness. Do not use soap on radiation fields, avoid direct sunlight, wind exposure, and washing with extremely cold/hot water or saline. For dry/itchy skin, apply menthol or talcum powder. Disinfectants like iodine or alcohol are prohibited in irradiated areas.

Maintain clear radiation field markings. Report fading to your radiation oncologist immediately for re-marking—never self-trace. Post-radiation skin burning/dryness/itching may occur—do not scratch. Male patients should use electric shavers to prevent skin damage. Maintain exact positioning without movement until treatment concludes.

2. Diet

Consume nutrient-dense, high-calorie foods: high-protein, high-vitamin, easily digestible options (eggs, fish, dairy). Eat fresh fruits/vegetables with diverse, balanced coarse/fine grains. Prioritize steaming, boiling, or stewing cooking methods. Avoid fried, grilled, coarse, spicy foods. Prevent nausea/vomiting by not eating 30 minutes before/after sessions. Practice food hygiene—avoid overeating, strong tea, coffee, greasy/spicy foods, and moldy items. Adopt small frequent meals. Increase water intake (2500-3000mL daily)

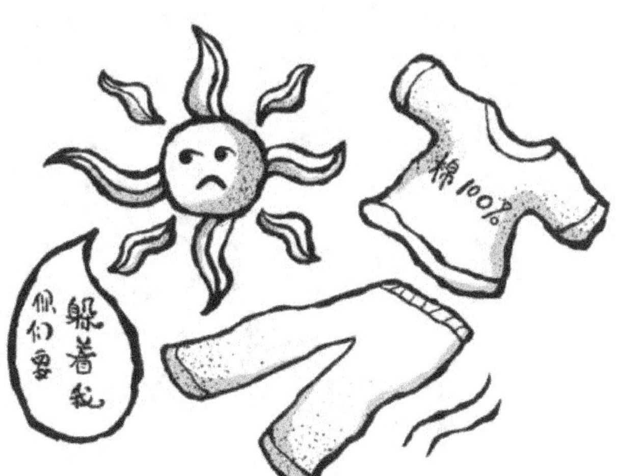

to flush radiotherapy metabolites. Monitor urine output.

Maintain oral hygiene: Rinse mouth frequently, brush morning/night, and rinse/brush after meals to remove food residues and reduce mucosal reactions.

3. Complication prevention guidance

(1) Systemic reactions: When radiotherapy is used to treat tumors, it not only destroys tumor cells, but also causes certain damage to normal tissues of the human body. Systemic reactions may occur 1 to 2 hours after irradiation, manifested as fatigue, nausea, vomiting, etc. If anorexia develops, avoid forced eating; use digestive aids to improve appetite.

(2) Myelosuppression: Myelosuppression may occur during large-area radiotherapy, leading to leukopenia. Patients should enhance nutrition, dress appropriately outdoors, and prevent infections.

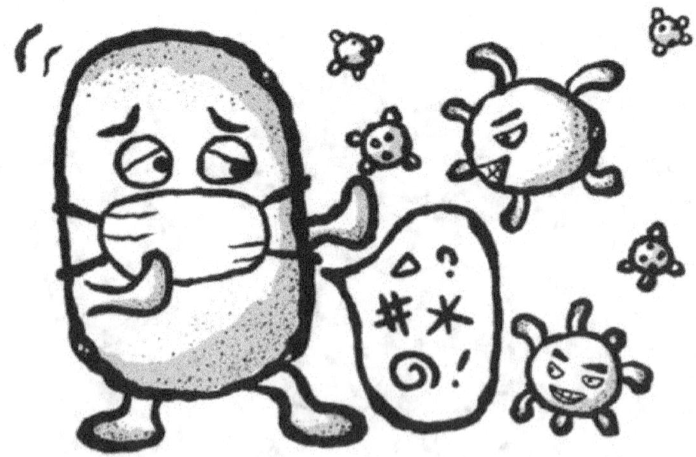

(3) Skin and mucosal reactions: Report redness/swelling/reduced saliva/dry mouth. Maintain oral cleanliness—avoid raw/cold/hard/irritating foods. Severe reactions require antibiotics and timed mouth rinsing. Pay attention to changes in the skin. If there is a burning or itching sensation, inform doctors and treat it in time.

(III) Post-radiotherapy

(1) Undergo a comprehensive examination after treatment completion, including blood count and X-ray examination, to monitor tumor status and radiotherapy side effects in a timely manner. Schedule annual checkups starting 3 months post-radiotherapy, including blood tests, MRI, X-rays, B-ultrasound, endoscopy, etc. (according to the specific requirements of doctors). Patients with abnormal blood counts during concurrent chemo-radiotherapy require weekly CBC/liver/kidney tests within 3 months after radiotherapy. Abnormal blood counts should be handled in a timely manner. Contact your doctor if you experience any discomfort.

(2) Pay attention to protecting the irradiated field skin, and follow medical instructions for radiation dermatitis. It is advisable to eat light and nourishing stews within 3 months post-treatment, such as light fish, chicken or lean pork with vegetables. Minimize fried, grilled, spicy, preserved and fatty foods. Engage in appropriate physical exercise such as jogging, table tennis, badminton, etc, according to patients' personal physical recovery. Intensity should feel comfortable post-activity. Return to work during

recovery, but increase rest time and avoid overexertion, heavy labor, night shifts, and high-altitude work, etc. Maintain a happy, optimistic and positive attitude.

(3) Head/neck radiotherapy patients are prohibited from having their teeth extracted or having dentures fitted within 3 years post-radiotherapy.

(4) Understand the adverse reactions of radiotherapy in detail, take preventive measures when necessary, and conduct regular reexaminations and follow-ups. Return to the hospital for reexamination one month after discharge, every three months within three years, and every six months after three years. Childbearing-age women must practice contraception; consulting their radiation oncologist before post-recovery pregnancy.

Patients often have different reactions during or after radiotherapy, so the precautions are also different.

3. Radiotherapy treatment sites

(I) Skin reactions

Common in breast cancer and head and neck malignancies, such as nasopharyngeal cancer, oral cancer, tongue cancer, pharyngeal cancer, and parotid cancer.

1. During treatment

Skin within radiation fields exhibits varying reactions according to dose and time. Generally, by the third or fourth week, redness, swelling, heat, and slight itching typically appear, resembling sunburned skin. Continued irradiation through the fifth or sixth week may darken skin color and cause dry desquamation. Some patients may develop wet desquamation.

2. Management methods

(1) Avoid washing or rubbing with soap.

(2) Do not apply ointments or makeup casually to avoid worsening skin reactions.

(3) For a slight itching sensation, refrain from scratching with nails to minimize irritation and skin breakdown. Use prescribed topical ointments only.

(4) Avoid exposure to sunlight.

(5) Prevent pressure, tight clothing, or friction from rough clothing.

(6) If unhealed wounds exist in treatment areas, physicians must evaluate before continuing treatment.

(7) For severe wet desquamation reaction, physicians will stop treatment

for 1 to 2 weeks or apply ointment depending on the situation, but do not apply it too thickly.

3. Post-treatment

(1) Avoid washing or rubbing the treated area with soap or irritating disinfectants. Wait until the skin has fully grown and recovered before washing it in the normal way.

(2) The darkening of skin color caused by treatment will fade away naturally.

(II) Head and neck treatment

1. Common reactions during treatment and management methods

(1) Oral mucositis: Typically appears around the third week of treatment. At this time, patients should avoid smoking, drinking, and sour/ spicy foods. Patients should often rinse their mouths with warm water or use mouthwashes and ointments prescribed by doctors.

(2) Dry mouth: Reduced saliva production due to irradiation causes dryness. Patients need to carry water for rinsing/drinking, use mouthwash prescribed by doctors to moisten the

mouth, take saliva-promoting Chinese medicine, and maintain a high indoor humidity.

(3) Mandibular joint ankylosis: Patients often develop tight jaw joints post-treatment, so they should start practicing mouth opening exercises during treatment.

(4) Taste dullness: Radiation to oral areas alters taste buds, reducing food flavor perception. When this phenomenon occurs, it is necessary to adjust food seasoning. Normal taste gradually recovers after treatment completion.

(5) Symptoms of intracranial hypertension include dizziness, worsening headache, nausea, projectile vomiting, and blurred vision. Common in whole-brain irradiation or patients with large lesions/severe cerebral edema, physicians will administer oral or infusion treatment to reduce intracranial pressure, depending on the situation.

2. Post-treatment

(1) Patients need to attend dental clinic regularly to monitor oral hygiene, dental caries, and lesions.

(2) Tooth extraction should be avoided as much as possible for 1–3 years after treatment completion. If tooth extraction is necessary, the decision should be made after careful examination by doctors.

(3) Radiation-induced otitis media: Radiation otitis media can cause ear pain, hearing loss, pus discharge, and even perforation of the eardrum. In this case, treat with

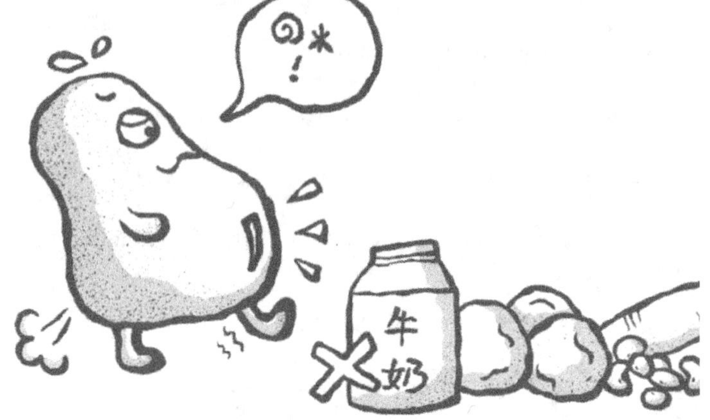

antibiotics, chloramphenicol in glycerol, or hydrogen peroxide ear drops to prevent/manage otitis media.

(III) Chest and upper abdomen treatment

1. Common reactions during treatment and management methods

(1) Nausea and vomiting: At this time, patients should consume bland, and easily digestible food, eat small meals frequently, and take prescription medicines from doctors in severe cases.

(2) Throat and esophageal pain: At this time, patients should consume cold, soft foods to alleviate pain and discomfort.

(3) Cough: This is caused by increased tracheal secretions during treatment and can be treated with prescription medication from physicians.

2. Post-treatment

Breast cancer patients may develop ipsilateral upper limb lymphedema due to axillary lymph node surgery and radiotherapy. After treatment completion, they need to maintain ongoing exercise and self-monitoring of the affected limb.

(IV) Lower abdominal treatment

Common for pelvic irradiation targeting rectal, bladder, and cervical malignancies.

1. Common reactions during treatment and management methods

(1) Abdominal pain, diarrhea, and bloating: These symptoms usually appear 2–3 weeks post-treatment initiation. Patients should consume bland, low-residue diets and avoid gas-producing foods such as beans or milk. Taking medication prescribed by physicians can also alleviate symptoms.

(2) Frank blood in stool or occult blood positivity is generally mild and can be managed with oral hemostatic drugs under medical guidance.

(3) Cystitis: Encourage drinking plenty of water and taking physician-prescribed medications.

2. Post-treatment

Patients with gynecological malignancies or inguinal irradiation often develop lower limb edema. When this occurs, it is recommended to avoid prolonged standing, elevate lower limbs during rest/sleep or wear compression stockings.

In addition, radiotherapy may cause granulocytopenia. During treatment, patients' immunity decreases, so it is necessary to avoid infection and enhance nutrition.

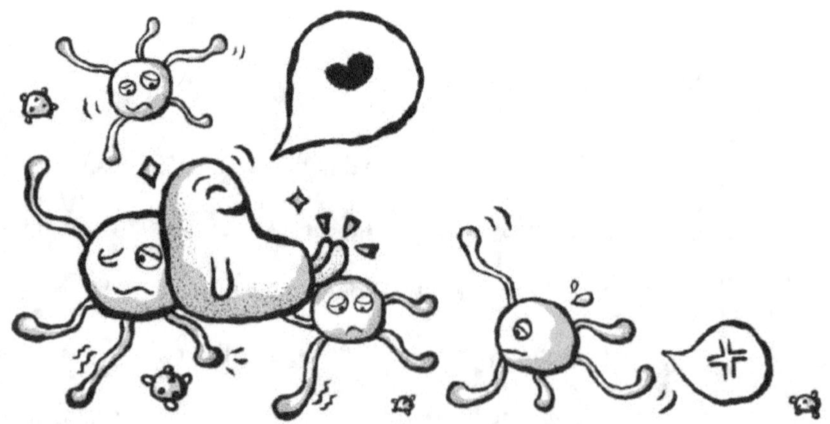

Part 14: Dietary Guidance During Radiotherapy

Radiotherapy patients often experience varying degrees of systemic reactions, gastrointestinal reactions, and bone marrow suppression reactions during treatment. If combined with appropriate nutritional therapy, it can not only ensure the smooth progress of radiotherapy, but also enhance efficacy while reducing side effects. Therefore, nutritional support is an important measure to maintain the physical strength and anti-cancer ability of radiotherapy patients and improve the efficacy.

1. Dietary principles for radiotherapy patients

Patients' diet should follow the principle of "three highs and one low": three highs refer to high vitamins, high proteins, and high calories, such as lean meat, seafood, fresh fruits, and vegetables; one low refers to low fat. Adequate hydration is essential. Additionally, patients should consume bland and easily digestible foods, avoid greasy and spicy items. Prepare meals to be palatable and appealing.

1. Dietary recommendations

(1) Choose foods with anti-cancer effects. Many bioactive substances exist in foods, such as lentinan, flavonoids, chlorophyll, lycopene, oryzanol, tea polyphenols, etc., which can prevent tumors and enhance immunity. These active compounds are predominantly found in plant-based foods like vegetables and fruits. Regularly consume raw and well-chewed tomatoes, cucumbers, radishes, carrots, red dates, hawthorns, grapes, apples, oranges, bananas, and walnuts. Additionally, increase intake of foods rich in trace

elements of selenium and molybdenum, such as mushrooms, fungus, kelp, garlic, onions, cabbage, corn, soybeans, lentils, radishes and dark-colored vegetables.

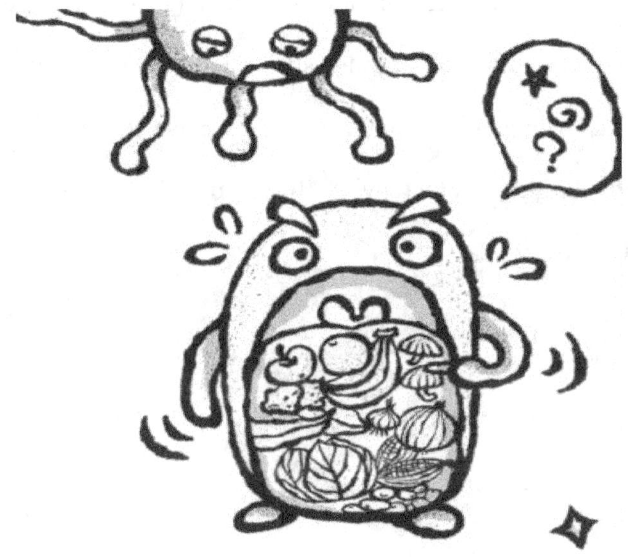

(2) Consume more mood-enhancing foods and potassium-rich foods like bananas, potatoes, spinach, etc.

(3) Eat foods that strengthen the spleen and stimulate appetite, such as coix seed, white lentils, yams, lotus seeds, red beans, jujubes, etc.

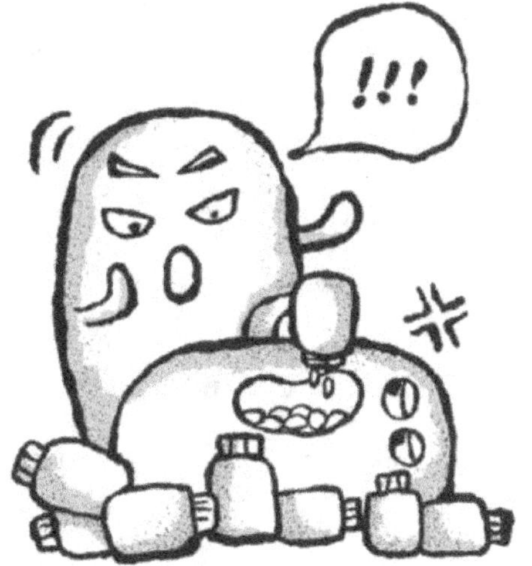

(4) Mild tea may be consumed in moderation.

(5) Drink plenty of water after radiotherapy, preferably between meals or 30 minutes before meals. Minimize or avoid drinking during meals. Adjust food choices based on radiotherapy reactions. For example, after leukopenia occurs, increase consumption of animal liver, spinach, and soy products. If patients experience anorexia or indigestion due to radiotherapy, adopt small frequent meals without reducing total intake. It is not recommended to avoid certain foods during radiotherapy. Daily vitamin C intake should reach no less than 1000 mg per day.

2. Dietary restrictions

(1) Avoid sudden intensive tonic intake to prevent gastrointestinal dysfunction, diarrhea, and anorexia.

(2) Refrain from long-term vegetarianism; do not blindly avoid so-called "trigger foods." Fresh fruits and vegetables are beneficial, but they cannot provide comprehensive nutrition.

(3) Avoid relying on health supplements.

(4) Hot-natured foods such as dog meat, lamb, as well as spices like chili, Sichuan pepper, black pepper, mustard, star anise, and cinnamon should be avoided or consumed sparingly.

(5) Quit smoking and drinking. Avoid cold water and refrain from eating salted, smoked, burnt, or moldy foods.

(6) Limit sweets, meats, and high-fat foods. Multivariate analysis results show that a high-fat diet is a risk factor for ovarian cancer in women.

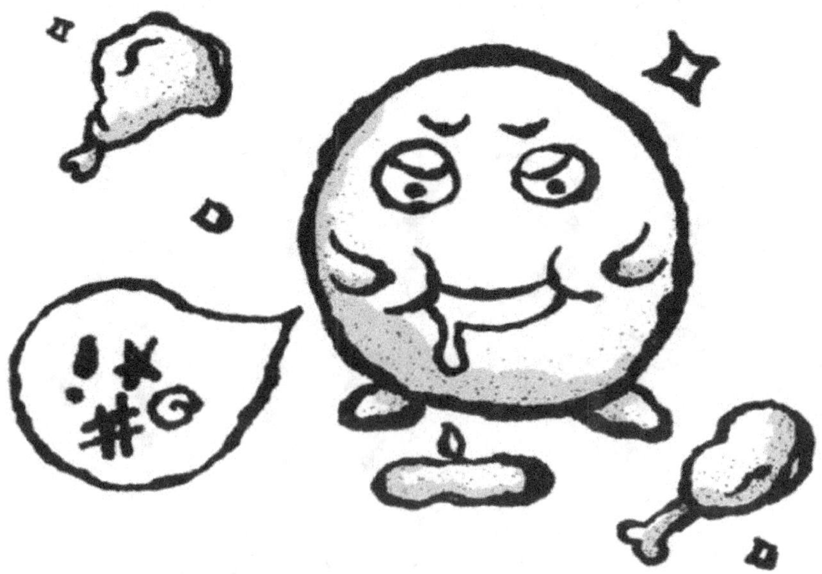

2. Dietary guidance during radiotherapy

Radiotherapy patients should consume high-protein, high-calorie diets with balanced animal and plant proteins. Prepare foods primarily by boiling, stewing, steaming, or braising. Avoid smoked, grilled, and fried foods.

1. Nutritional preparation one week before radiotherapy

The primary goal is to enhance physical constitution. Increase intake of lean meat, chicken, duck, eggs, milk, aquatic products (fish), soy products, rice, noodles, grains, fresh vegetables and fruits, etc., specifically high in protein (increase by 50%), high in calories (increase by 20%, no increase for obese people), and high in vitamins, so that the body has a certain nutritional reserve. Foods that replenish Qi, blood, spleen and kidney, such as red dates, yams, sesame, beef, soy products, fish, eggs and milk, etc.

2. During radiotherapy

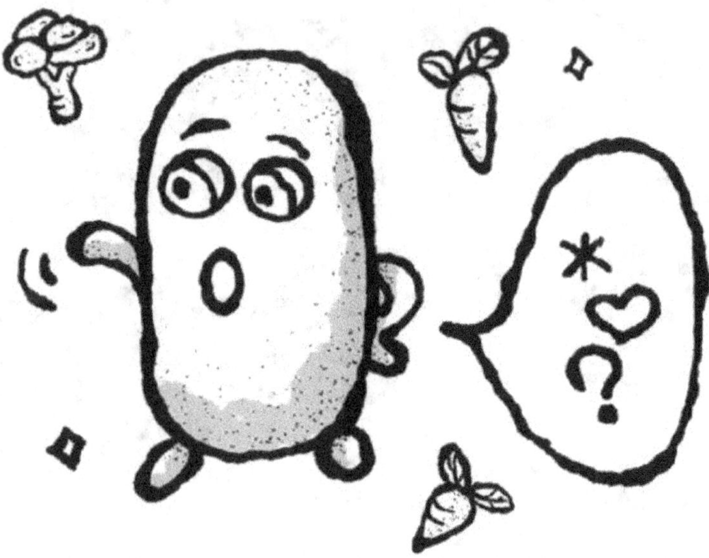

Significantly increase soup-based dishes, tea, and beverages to ensure adequate hydration. Beyond food moisture, supplement with over 2000mL daily. In addition, patients should eat more porridge, vegetable soup, watermelon, tofu brain, mung bean soup, soy milk, fruit and vegetable juice, etc.

Radiotherapy often causes "internal heat". Heating-nature foods such as dog meat, mutton, chili peppers, Sichuan peppercorns, black pepper, mustard, star anise, and cinnamon bark should be avoided or minimized. Salted, smoked, burnt, and moldy foods should not be consumed. It is better to eat fresh food, diversify the food, and pay attention to nutritional balance.

3. Symptomatic dietary management during radiotherapy

(I) Gastrointestinal reactions

1. Anorexia

When severe gastrointestinal reactions occur during radiotherapy, it is advisable to choose nutritious, light and easy-to-digest semi-liquid food, liquid food, clear liquid and other soft food. Such as various vegetable porridge, fine noodles, wontons, etc., or a nutritionally balanced nutrient solution. Increase salt intake moderately. Excessively sweet or greasy foods may further reduce appetite and should be avoided.

2. Nausea and vomiting

It is more common during radiotherapy for abdominal tumors. The diet should be light and less greasy, eat small meals frequently, add a small amount of ginger juice to the dishes for seasoning, avoid stale protein foods and other foods with strange smells. Patients can also eat fresh ginger slices. Huoxiang ZhengQi liquid can reduce gastrointestinal reactions. Prefer finely textured foods; yogurt may replace milk.

Huoxiang Zhengqi Liquid, Banxia Shumi congee, and ginger juice are highly effective in relieving nausea and vomiting. For severe vomiting, patients may slowly chew and swallow ice chips or consume fresh vitamin C-rich juices.

Patients should avoid eating within 1 hour before radiotherapy. Select bland foods, avoid overly sweet or greasy items, and refrain from consuming large volumes of fluids at once. Do not mix hot and cold foods. Maintain a calm eating environment to stabilize mood and enhance comfort.

3. Abdominal distension and diarrhea

Caused by accelerated intestinal peristalsis due to radiation-induced mucosal irritation. At this time, it is advisable to consume easily digestible, light, and less greasy foods, such as semi-liquid diets or diets with less residue. Avoid foods high in fiber and sticky, cold foods. Eat less gas-producing foods, such as beans, milk, and carbonated drinks. When the abdominal distension reaction occurs, patients can massage their abdomen after meals to relieve this symptom.

4. Constipation

Some radiotherapy patients may experience constipation. They should increase physical activity moderately and consume more fresh vegetables, fruits, and other foods rich in fiber, such as bananas, apples, potatoes, sweet potatoes, etc. Take a cup of honey water before going to bed every night. Consider Chinese medicine Ma Ren Run Chang Wan or a small amount of liquid paraffin if necessary.

(II) Dry mouth, sore throat, and esophagitis

These are the most common radiation reactions in patients with head, neck or chest tumors and are caused by radiation damage to the salivary glands and mucosa. Adopt small frequent meals. For severe symptoms, hold or swallow small amounts of tetracaine or lidocaine solution before eating to significantly reduce pain.

(III) Altered taste

Radiotherapy usually reduces sensitivity to sweet/sour tastes while increasing bitterness perception. Sugar or lemon can enhance sweetness and sourness, so use more of them when cooking, and avoid consuming foods with a strong bitter taste, such as mustard greens. Patients can choose foods with stronger flavors, use sugar or lemon to enhance sweetness and sourness, and choose foods with unique flavors such as mushrooms and onions. Minimize bitter melon or mustard greens. Adjust the amount of salt according to patients' feelings. Using cold dishes with appropriate seasonings will be attractive to cancer patients with altered taste.

(IV) Frequent urination, urgency, pain during urination, and hematuria

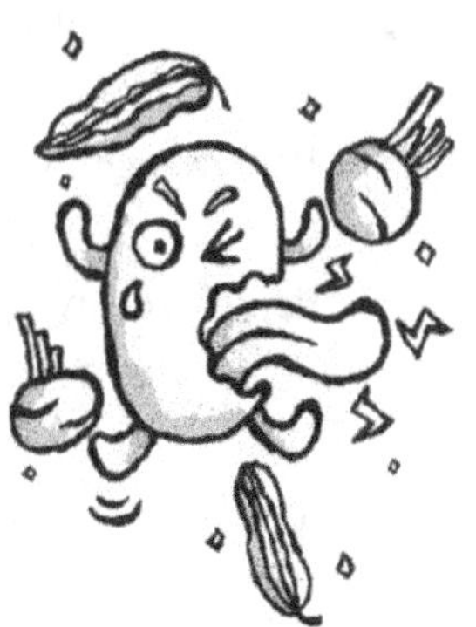

This is a symptom of radiation cystitis, which often occurs during or after radiotherapy for pelvic tumors such as bladder cancer, prostate cancer, and cervical cancer. Increase fluid intake and urination frequency. Administer sodium bicarbonate to alkalinize urine.

(V) Myelosuppression

During leukopenia/thrombocytopenia, it is advisable to provide high-protein and iron-rich foods. While using Western hematinic drugs, supplement with blood-enhancing medicated diets (Codonopsis root, astragalus, Chinese angelica, cooked rehmannia, peanuts, red dates, red beans, partridge eggs). If conditions are available, patients can have some tonics such as American ginseng, royal jelly, Poria, wolfberry, deer antler and other Chinese medicines may be used as blood/qi tonics.

4. Dietary guidance after radiotherapy for different cancer patients

1. Patients with head tumors

Prone to mucosal ulcers, mastication and swallowing difficulties. Prioritize yin-nourishing, brain-tonifying, and mind-calming foods. The diet should consist of bland, low-fat, non-irritating, easy-to-chew semi-liquid food and soft rice, and increase the supply of vitamin A and vitamin C.

2. Patients with neck tumors

Patients receiving radiotherapy to neck/esophageal areas may experience decreased or absent sense of taste, decreased saliva secretion, dry mouth, mucosal ulcers, and difficulty chewing and swallowing. Consume finely textured semi-liquid or homogenized diets. The temperature of the food should not be too cold or too hot to reduce the stimulation to the lesion. At the same time, they can swallow warm water before and after eating to reduce the adhesion of food to the lesion. Avoid eating salty, spicy, strong-flavored, rough and hard food. Maintain oral hygiene before and after meals. Emphasize heat-clearing, fire-reducing, yin-nourishing, and fluid-promoting foods such as watermelon, pear, orange, grapefruit, apple, lemon, lotus root, water chestnut, bitter melon, wild rice stem, cabbage, green tea, honey, crucian carp, jellyfish, mussels, bean soup, etc.

3. Patients with chest tumors

Prioritize yin-nourishing, lung-moistening, phlegm-dissolving, cough-relieving foods including winter melon, watermelon, loofah, cucumber, orange, pear, loquat, apricot, plum, lotus root, yam, carrot, eel, etc. Patients with lung cancer must exercise particular caution with irritating foods.

4. Patients with abdominal tumors

Patients can choose foods that strengthen the spleen and stomach, nourish blood and replenish Qi, such as bayberry, hawthorn, orange, tangerine, chicken gizzard, goose blood, coix seed, fresh ginger, etc. Abdominal radiotherapy may cause nausea and vomiting in some patients. Consume light, low-fat foods in small frequent portions. Add minimal ginger juice to dishes for flavor enhancement.

5. Patients with urogenital tumors

Patients can choose kidney-tonifying, liver-nourishing, yin-cultivating, heat-clearing foods including figs, watermelon, bitter gourd, cucumber, coriander, pepper, fennel, placenta, milk, eggs, sunflower seeds, etc.

Part 15: Common Toxic Side Effects of Radiotherapy and Brief Treatment and Nursing Care

1. Radiation dermatitis

Inflammatory damage to the skin and mucous membranes caused by ionizing radiation. It is one of the common complications induced by radiotherapy. This condition primarily occurs in patients undergoing radiation therapy and radiation workers with inadequate protection. It may cause a series of skin reactions and injuries, manifesting as reversible hair loss, dermatitis, pigmentation and irreversible skin atrophy, destruction of sebaceous glands and sweat glands and permanent hair loss, resulting in radiation necrosis and subsequent ulcer formation.

(I) Clinical manifestations

1. Clinical manifestations of acute radiation skin injury

Acute radiation skin injury is generally classified into four degrees:

Degree I: Dry desquamation, pigmentation, subjective burning sensation.

Degree II: Tender bright erythema, moist peeling, moderate edema, pain. After eschar detachment, hyperpigmentation remains without scar formation.

Degree III: Develop after patchy edematous erythema, moist peeling outside the skin folds, pitting edema, and increased pain.

Degree IV (Ulceration): severe pain, bleeding, necrosis, involving the dermis, muscles, and even bones.

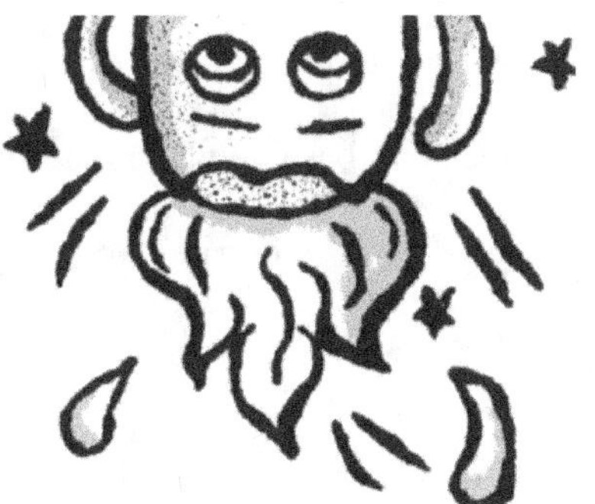

2. Clinical manifestations of chronic radiation skin injury

There is a long incubation period, and the disease is characterized by obvious latent, progressive, recurrent and persistent characteristics. It is divided into four types: chronic radiation dermatitis (the most common), indurated edema, chronic radiation ulcer and radiation-induced skin cancer.

(1) Chronic radiation dermatitis: Skin atrophy with degeneration/loss of glands and hair follicles; dry, inelastic skin; alternating pigmentation and depigmentation, thinned epidermis, superficial telangiectasia; desquamation; pruritus.

(2) Induration edema: The local skin becomes swollen and thickened, with an orange-peel texture and board-like hardness. The edema spreads to the subcutaneous tissue and is very easy to rupture.

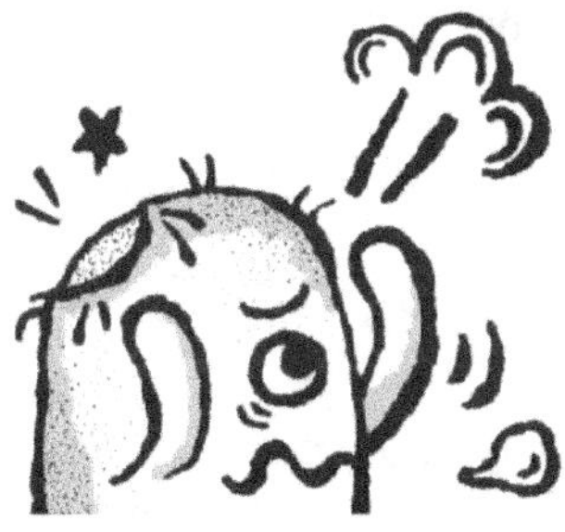

(3) Chronic radiation ulcers: The wound surface is dirty and pale, with varying degrees of infection, and the area around the ulcer shows radiation dermatitis.

(4) Radiation-induced skin cancer: Predominantly squamous cell carcinoma and basal cell carcinoma. Sarcoma, melanoma and sebaceous gland carcinoma occurring on the basis of chronic dermatitis have been reported.

(II) Treatment

Includes conservative therapy, surgical intervention, and physical therapy.

1. Conservative therapy

(1) Degree I:

Exposure therapy and use Kangyongte ointment, Biafen ointment or Saifurun spray to apply to the radiotherapy area.

(2) Degree II:

Exposure therapy and use Kangyongte ointment, Bifen ointment or Saifurun spray to apply to the radiotherapy area. For ruptured blisters, use a mixture of silver sulfadiazine ointment and recombinant human epidermal growth factor gel mixed and applied.

(3) Degree III:

After cleaning the wound with saline, apply a mixture of silver sulfadiazine ointment and recombinant human epidermal growth factor gel to prevent infection. If necessary, perform bacterial culture from the wound and use appropriate antibiotics for symptomatic treatment.

(4) Degree IV:

Administer anti-infection treatment, debride, and perform skin grafting if indicated.

2. Surgical treatment

For non-healing ulcers with necrosis, surgical intervention should be performed as soon as possible once infection has subsided, provided the patient's overall condition permits.

3. Physical therapy

(1) High-flow oxygen therapy: Accelerates wound healing via localized tissue oxygenation.

(2) Laser treatment

(III) Nursing

1. Psychological support

Observe patients' emotional changes in a timely manner when their skin reacts. Listen patiently to patients' concerns and thoroughly explain the relevant radiotherapy knowledge and its significance.

2. Local skin care

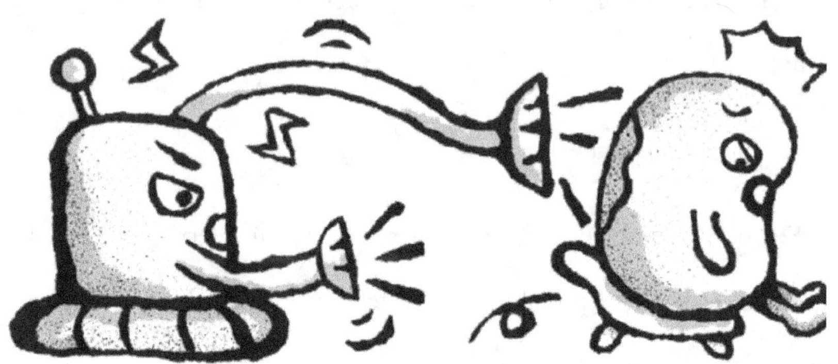

(1) Skin protection

(i) Select loose, soft, and highly absorbent cotton undergarments;

(ii) Keep the irradiated area dry. Clean gently without scrubbing. Prohibit soap, shower gel, etc., do not use irritating disinfectants such as iodine oil, alcohol cosmetics, etc., and avoid hot and cold stimulation such as hot compresses, ice packs, etc.;

(iii) Do not apply ointments, creams, or lotions to irradiated areas unless prescribed by a radiation oncologist;

(iv) Remove watches, jewelry, and dentures before entering the radiation room, as heavy metals can produce secondary radiation and aggravate radiation damage to the skin;

(v) Avoid temperature extremes and direct sunlight on the irradiated area;

(vi) Do not scratch, tear or peel the skin when it is flaking. Refrain from shaving hair in irradiated zones. Use razors to prevent skin infection. Maintain skin cleanliness and dryness. Apply skin protectants before and after radiation.

(vii) Keep the irradiation field marks clearly visible.

(2) Promoting skin reaction healing

(i) Dry reactions: Implement exposure therapy.

(ii) Moist reactions: Implement exposure therapy, keep the local area dry, and use medication as prescribed by doctors. If ulcers have scabbed, the scab cannot be removed by hand, and it should be allowed to fall off naturally to avoid combined infection.

(3) Diet care

(i) Strengthening nutrition can promote tissue repair. Consume high-energy, high-protein, vitamin-rich and easily digestible foods. For patients with poor appetite, administer intravenous nutrition to maintain fluid-electrolyte and acid-base balance.

(ii) Create a safe, clean and comfortable dining environment for patients and encourage them to drink more water.

3. Health education

To reduce the severity of skin reactions, preventive skin care measures should be emphasized at the beginning of treatment to protect the irradiated skin and prevent skin reactions.

(1) Undergarments should be soft, loose, and highly absorbent. The collar and edges of the clothes should not be too hard to avoid friction with rough clothing.

(2) Keep high-perspiration skin areas such as the armpits, under the breasts, groin, and vulva clean and dry to prevent dry reactions progressing to moist reactions;

(3) The irradiation field can be gently washed with warm water and soft towels. Soap is not allowed to be used to scrub the local area. Avoid hot and cold stimulation such as hot compresses, hot water bottles, ice bags, etc. Prohibit iodine, alcohol and other irritating disinfectants. Do not apply ointments and other irritating drugs;

(4) Heavy metals such as zinc oxide can produce secondary radiation that aggravates skin damage, so adhesive tape should not be applied within the irradiation field;

(5) Shield skin from direct sunlight when outdoors;

(6) The irradiated skin is prohibited from being shaved. An electric shaver is recommended to prevent skin damage and infection. The irradiated

skin is prohibited from being used as an injection site.

(7) Avoid scratching. Never manually peel desquamated skin. Hair follicles are sensitive to radiation, so patients with head tumors should be informed of the possibility of hair loss before further irradiation, but hair can regenerate 2 to 3 months after stopping radiotherapy. During radiotherapy, increase hydration to eliminate toxins and eat high-protein, high-vitamin foods, such as spinach, leeks, tomatoes and other fruits and vegetables, as well as soybeans, walnuts, peanuts and other shelled foods.

(IV) Discharge guidance

Protect irradiated skin for ≥1 month post-treatment.

Follow-up guidance should be maintained once a week during the period after radiotherapy and one month after discharge. Medical staff will timely monitor the progression and recovery of the patients' radiation-induced dermatitis, and instruct the patients to keep the irradiated skin clean, dry, and prevent infection and avoid irritation during the recovery period. Adhere strictly to the "four prohibitions, four bans, one avoidance and one refrain" principle:

(1) Four prohibitions:

Do not scratch/rub skin;

Do not wear stiff high-collared clothing (for neck irradiation);

Do not expose to intense sunlight;

Do not undergo infrared lamp therapy;

Four bans:

Ban adhesive tapes/patches;

Ban injections;

Ban heat application;

Ban self-medication;

One avoidance:

Avoid washing with soap or skin cream

One refrain:

Refrain from applying irritants or

heavy metal-containing drugs, such as iodine, mercurochrome, balm,

etc.

2. Adiation-induced oral mucositis

Radiation-induced oral mucositis refers to inflammation of oral and intraoral soft tissues caused by ionizing radiation damage to oral mucosal cells during radiotherapy, resulting in oral ulcers and infection. It is a common side effect of radiotherapy for head and neck tumors. Severe mucosal reactions often reduce patients' food/fluid intake, leading to fluid-electrolyte imbalances, acid-base imbalance and malnutrition. Incidence reaches 85%–100% in head/neck cancer patients undergoing conventional radiotherapy or concurrent chemoradiation.

(I) Clinical manifestations

The development of oral mucositis can be divided into three stages: initial, peak and persistence.

The chance of oral infection is greatly increased due to damage to the oral mucosa and decreased immunity caused by radiotherapy and chemotherapy.

Categorized into acute and chronic radiation-induced oral mucositis.

1. Clinical manifestations of acute radiation oral mucositis

Develops during or within 6 months post-radiation. Presents as mucosal erythema, edema, patchy mucositis, and scattered soft white elevated spots. Spots coalesce into white patches with inflammatory/hemorrhagic exudate, ulcers, and pain. Systemic symptoms include fatigue, dizziness, nausea, and insomnia.

2. Clinical manifestations of chronic radiation oral mucositis

Either persists from acute mucositis or emerges >6 months post-radiation. Features mucosal atrophy, variably deep ulcers with poor healing, and recurrent episodes. Dominant symptoms: salivary gland atrophy and xerostomia.

(II) Treatment

The principle is to alleviate symptoms, promote mucosal healing, and restore oral function. Approaches include analgesia, anti-infection, and the use of cytoprotective agents. Immunocompromised or debilitated patients require systemic supportive care.

1. Pain relief: The most commonly used method of pain relief is to use procaine as a basic local anesthesia. For those who are affected by pain in eating and sleeping, local anesthetics can be used as gargles to relieve pain, or pain relief drugs can be used before meals or sleep.

2. Anti-infection: Medication under medical supervision.

3. Cytoprotective agents: Cytoprotectants can be divided into direct cytoprotectants and indirect cytoprotectants.

Direct cytoprotectants include sucralfate, glutathione, β-carotene, vitamin E, vitamin C, prostaglandins (PGE2) and hormones (betamethasone), etc.

Indirect cytoprotectants include granulocyte colony stimulating factor (G-CSF), granulocyte-macrophage colony stimulating factor (GM-CSF) and epidermal growth factor (EGF). Traditional chinese medicine (TCM): Yin deficiency and heat-toxicity are core pathogenesis. Therefore, clearing away heat and detoxifying, nourishing yin and promoting fluid production are the most common treatment principles for radiation oral mucositis.

4. Other therapies

(1) Oral cryotherapy: Currently, a more effective preventive measure, which can reduce the incidence of oral

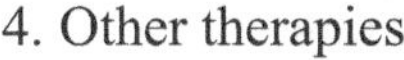

mucositis by about 50%.

(2) Helium-neon laser: Reduce the severity of mucositis and pain, improve swallowing function.

(III) Nursing

1. Prevention

Preventing the occurrence of oral mucositis can improve quality of life during radiotherapy/chemotherapy. Emphasizing mouthwash and taking oral care measures to reduce the occurrence of oral mucositis.

(1) Gum and oral inflammation should be treated before radiotherapy and chemotherapy. Perform prophylactic dental cleaning. Avoid dental procedures during treatment.

(2) Maintain oral moisture. Carry drinking water and encourage >2500 mL/day intake. Patients can soak honeysuckle and ophiopogon japonicus in water and take them orally to moisten the oral mucosa.

(3) Maintain oral hygiene. Brush with a soft-bristle toothbrush and non-irritating toothpaste. Rinse pre/post meals with mild saline (500 mL of warm water plus 3-4 g of salt), compound boric acid solution, dobell's solution, 3% sodium bicarbonate, or 3% hydrogen peroxide to keep the mouth clean and moist.

(4) Avoid tobacco, alcohol, and irritating foods: Excessively hot/cold, hard, spicy, coarse-textured items.

(5) Patients should chew gum frequently and do more chewing exercises to alleviate the difficulty in opening the mouth.

(6) Actively treat upper respiratory and paranasal sinus infections.

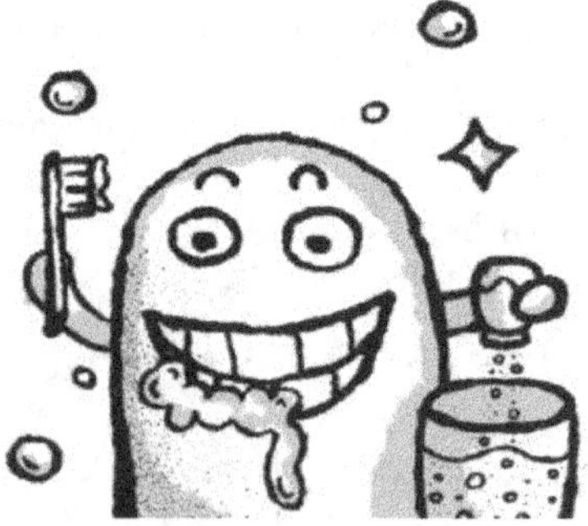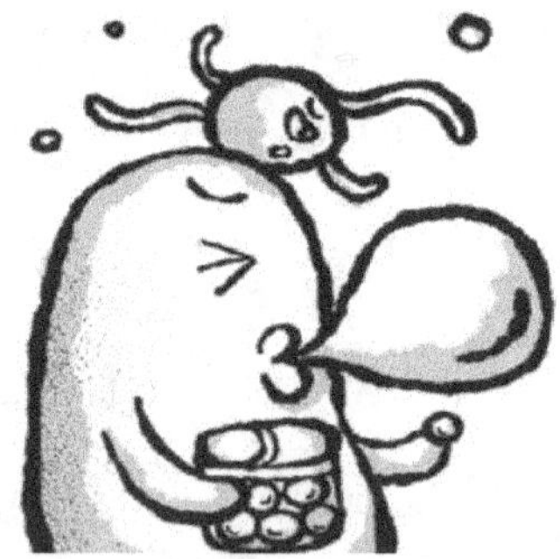

2. Nursing

(1) Prior to radiotherapy, perform dental cleaning and address oral pathologies: Repair of shallow caries, removal of metal braces, extraction of deep caries and residual roots, treatment of apical periodontitis, gingivitis, etc. Initiate radiotherapy only after wound healing (approximately 7–10 days).

(2) Close observation: Daily meticulous assessment of oral mucosa. Patients with oral diseases must receive treatment first.

(3) When oral mucositis occurs, provide active symptomatic care and guide patients to use local medications correctly to achieve the best results.

(i) Grade I oral mucositis: mucosal congestion, edema, and mild pain.

Advise patients against spicy, fried, rough, overcold, overheated, hard and other irritating foods. Increase fresh vegetables, fruits rich in vitamins and fluid intake (2000–2500mL/day). Drink water soaked with honeysuckle, chrysanthemum, licorice, ophiopogon, etc.

Maintain oral hygiene: Rinse before and after meals, and brush teeth with a soft-bristled toothbrush. Patients may use mouthwash or Kangfuxin

solution for rinsing. For sensitivity, use warm water gargles. Perform oral rinses at 40-60 minute intervals with cheek puffing. For mouthwash use: administer 10-20 ml per rinse, retain in oral cavity for at least 2 to 5 minutes, then expel (do not swallow).

For those with mild oral edema, rinse the mouth with sodium bicarbonate to improve oral pH.

Nebulize with 0.9% normal saline 10 mL+ chymotrypsin 40 million U+ dexamethasone 5 mg to deliver medication directly to the oropharyngeal mucosa, reducing patients' oral mucosal damage.

Dexamethasone: It can reduce local mucosal exudation, edema, capillary dilation, phagocytic reaction of leukocyte infiltration and other inflammatory reactions.

Chymotrypsin: Cleaves secretions for easier expulsion, maintaining cleanliness.

Lidocaine: It can paralyze the sensory endings under the mucosa and

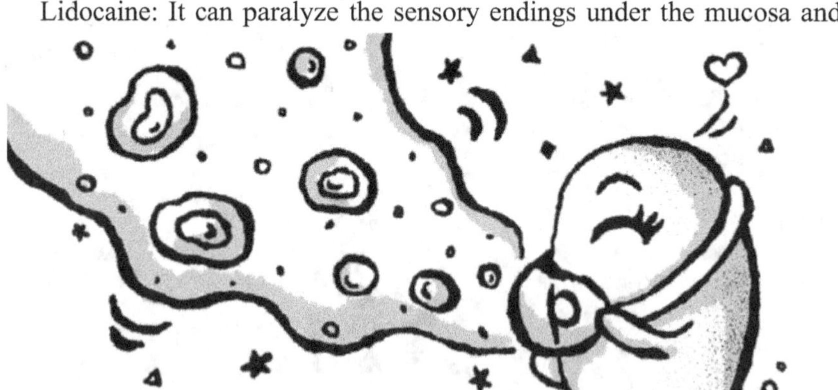

have an analgesic effect.

Honeysuckle and Ophiopogon japonicus: Traditional Chinese Medicine discipline believes that honeysuckle and Ophiopogon japonicus could clear away heat and promote the production of body fluids, increase saliva secretion, and accelerate the healing of ulcers. Therefore, meticulous oral care and rational use of drugs can reduce acute mucosal reactions, relieve oral pain, and enable patients to successfully complete the course of treatment.

(ii) Grade II oral mucositis: Mucosal congestion and edema, macular ulcers or pseudomembrane formation, and moderate pain.

A. Sustain oral cleanliness.

B. Nebulize twice daily with 0.9% saline 10 mL+ chymotrypsin 1 vial+ dexamethasone 5 mg, or select sensitive drugs according to the results of drug sensitivity test;

C. Homemade rinse: 0.9% saline 500 mL+ 2% lidocaine 10 mL+ vitamin B12 40 mg. Hold 10–20mL orally thrice daily. Local spraying of Kangfuxin promotes cell maturation and release, repairs damaged cells, and helps repair oral mucosal ulcers.

D. Guide patients to eat high-protein, high-vitamin liquid or semi-liquid diets. Supplement with water-soluble vitamins intravenously.

(iii) Grade III oral mucositis: Mucosal congestion, edema, confluent ulcers or pseudomembrane formation; bleeding caused by non-minor trauma, and pain that seriously affects eating.

A. Rinse the mouth frequently, once every 30 minutes, to keep the mouth clean. Patients can choose a suitable mouthwash based on the results of throat swab culture or oral pH value.

B. Follow doctors' instructions for anti-infection treatment and oral care. First, scrub the mouth with a saline-soaked cotton ball, and then gargle with mouthwash for 5 to 10 minutes.

C. Use drugs that promote mucosal healing, such as Jinyin peptide, Kangfuxin, etc. If the pain of an oral ulcer affects patients' eating, use a mouthwash containing anesthetics such as lidocaine for 2 to 3 minutes, 5–10 minutes pre-meal. Avoid rinsing/drinking before eating to retain the local concentration of the drug, reduce the pain caused by eating stimulation.

D. According to the three-step pain relief principle, administer painkillers if needed, monitor side effects and provide relevant health education at the same time.

E. Consider antibiotics and intravenous nutritional support or nasogastric feeding if necessary.

(iv) Grade IV oral mucositis: large-area ulcers of the mucosa, tissue necrosis: severe pain that makes it impossible to eat, obvious spontaneous bleeding, and life-threatening complications.

A. Suspend radiotherapy.

B. Administer painkillers.

C. Perform oral care with 0.9% saline to clean the secretions, encourage patients to rinse the mouth more frequently, and monitor the changes of the ulcer. Apply Yunnan Baiyao locally for hemostasis.

D. Initiate antibiotics or antifungal drugs for treatment.

E. Supportive treatments such as nasogastric feeding, intravenous hypernutrition, and albumin supplementation.

F. Monitor vital signs, electrolytes and blood routine.

(4) Psychological support: Address anxiety, depression, and pessimism common in cancer patients. In addition, prolonged treatment and severe mucositis intensify fear. Most patients are afraid of radiotherapy. If severe stomatitis occurs during the irradiation process, it will affect patients' eating and rest, further increasing their psychological burden. In this regard, it is advisable to educate the basic knowledge of this disease and the therapeutic effect of radiotherapy on the disease to alleviate patients' distress and build their confidence.

(5) Nutritional support: Enhance immunity. Provide high-protein, high-vitamin, high-calorie diets. Avoid eating too cold, too hot, too hard, or fried foods. Avoid spicy and irritating foods. Adopt small frequent meals. At the same time, abstain from tobacco/alcohol. For patients with severe infection, fever, significant increase in white blood cells, and difficulty eating, initiate

systemic therapy.

3. Health education

(1) Instruct patients to remove dentures and inspect the oral cavity twice daily using a penlight and tongue depressor, monitoring for any abnormalities. Report any changes promptly to physicians or nurses.

(2) Brush teeth with a soft-bristled toothbrush half an hour after meals and every four hours. Soak the toothbrush in hot water to soften it before brushing, and brush with cooled boiled water. If patients are afraid that the toothbrush may sting the wound, patients can use a small wooden stick wrapped with gauze or a cotton swab to brush their teeth. After brushing, wash the toothbrush thoroughly and place it in a cool and dry place.

(3) Use non-irritating toothpaste or a baking soda solution for brushing.

(4) Before and after meals and before going to bed, rinse the mouth with a 1:3 mixture of mild saline or hydrogen peroxide (3%) and water.

(5) Keep lips moist. Consume at least 2 L of water or juice every day unless contraindicated.

(6) Consume bland and non-irritating foods, supplement with high-protein foods and vitamins. Adopt small frequent meals without excessive dietary restrictions.

(7) Do not extract teeth within 3 years after radiotherapy to prevent the

occurrence of radiation osteomyelitis.

(8) After the end of radiotherapy, patients may experience oral mucosal reactions such as pharyngeal and throat pain, swollen and painful gums, and thick sputum, which will last for 2 to 3 weeks. Instruct patients to continue frequent light salt or warm water gargles and to initiate anti-infection treatment when necessary. If symptoms are severe, seek medical attention in a timely manner. Oral mucosal reactions will gradually heal over time.

(9) For xerostomia: Patients can use tongue exercises to stimulate saliva secretion. The method is: move the tongue forward and backward, left and right, up and down in the mouth for 3 to 5 minutes each time, 3 times a day; patients can do more swallowing and chewing exercises to stimulate the salivary glands, prevent gland atrophy, and promote saliva secretion. The sense of taste will gradually recover 1 to 3 months post-treatment. If the dry mouth lasts for a long time, patients can drink a small amount of water frequently to maintain oral moisture.

(IV) Discharge guidance

Lifelong follow-up monitoring is mandatory. Patients should return to the hospital for a follow-up visit one month post-discharge. During the first three years post-radiotherapy, schedule quarterly evaluations. After three years, patients will conduct biannual assessments. A comprehensive examination should be conducted at the 3rd month, 6th month, and 1st year post-radiotherapy, and annually thereafter. This includes blood tests, magnetic resonance imaging (MRI), X-rays, ultrasound, and other assessments, as determined by the treating physician's specific requirements.

3. Radiation pneumonitis

Radiation pneumonitis is an inflammatory reaction in normal lung tissue within the radiation field after treatment for lung, mediastinum, tumor, esophageal cancer, breast cancer, malignant lymphoma or other parts of the chest. Mild cases may resolve without symptoms; severe cases can cause widespread lung fibrosis, leading to breathing problems or even respiratory failure.

(I) Clinical manifestations

The development of typical radiation pneumonitis can be divided into 4 stages:

Mild cases: Low-grade fever with occasional cough or chest tightness.

1. Moderate cases: Patients may experience breathing difficulties, chest pain, and persistent dry cough, sometimes with white or blood-streaked mucus.

2. Severe radiation pneumonitis: The main clinical manifestations are acute respiratory distress, high fever, and life-threatening complications.

3. Clinical symptoms are not specific. Early symptoms are often subtle, generally a mild cough, with a small amount of foamy sputum, typically

appearing 4 to 6 weeks after radiotherapy. Severe symptoms include cough, chest tightness, chest pain, dyspnea and fever. An irritating cough may start immediately after radiotherapy. Most symptoms appear 2 to 3 months after radiotherapy. Some patients may develop an irritating dry cough half a year after treatment, worsening with activity and accompanied by palpitations. Fever ranges from absent/low-grade to sudden high spikes.

4. Pulmonary function tests help detect early changes from lung inflammation or scarring.

(II) Treatment

Once diagnosed with radiation pneumonitis, patients should stop the radiotherapy as soon as possible.

1. Glucocorticoids therapy: Glucocorticoids therapy is the first choice for radiation pneumonitis.

2. Application of antibiotics: Radiation pneumonia is very likely to be complicated by bacterial infection. If high fever, increased white blood cell count and neutrophil count, and coughing up yellow sputum occur, sufficient and effective broad-spectrum antibiotics should be given at the same time as glucocorticoids, which can be effective more quickly.

3. Non-steroidal drugs: Indomethacin and aspirin can alleviate the clinical symptoms of radiation pneumonitis and play an auxiliary role.

4. Symptomatic supportive treatment: Oxygen inhalation and

increased nutrition, etc.

(III) Nursing

1. Prevention: Since prevention is paramount for radiation pneumonitis, especially in high-risk patients (elderly, children, those with diabetes or chronic lung disease), close monitoring is essential. This includes tracking temperature, heart rate, sputum characteristics, and lung signs, while paying particular attention to breathing rate and depth. Should any abnormalities arise, prompt treatment is crucial to prevent disease progression.

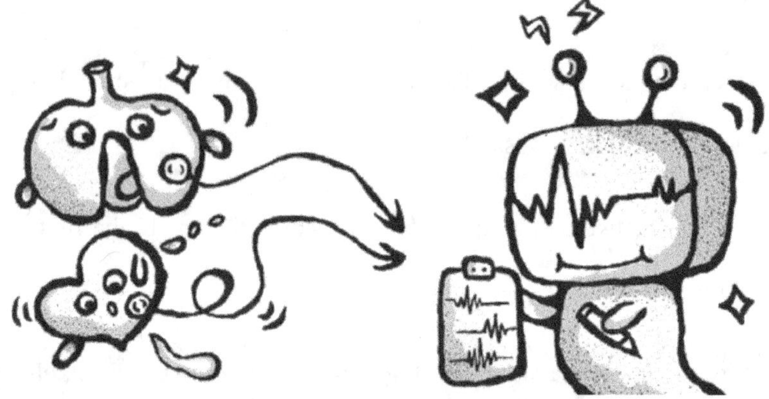

2. Cough management: Given that cough is a common symptom of radiation pneumonia. The pattern and timing of patients' cough, as well as the presence of concomitant symptoms such as hemoptysis and chest tightness, should be observed. Under medical guidance, antitussives may be used. For patients struggling with expectoration, perform back percussion and administer humidification or nebulization therapy when necessary to facilitate mucus clearance.

3. Dyspnea intervention: When patients experience dyspnea, they should be placed in a semi-recumbent position immediately. Oxygen should be administered at a flow rate of (2-4) L/min while guiding relaxed breathing techniques. Continuously monitor respiratory rate, rhythm, and depth throughout the episode.

4. Fever control: Fever is one of the main symptoms of lung cancer patients. Observe patients' body temperature changes. If it exceeds 39°C, initiate physical cooling. Maintain oral hygiene and hydration by encouraging frequent water intake.

5. Daily living support: Ensure adequate rest with bed confinement during acute phases. Provide easily digestible, high-protein/high-calorie liquid or semi-liquid meals (e.g., nutrient shakes, pureed vegetables) to sustain nutritional needs.

6. Ward requirements: Open windows and doors regularly for ventilation, keep the room clean and the air fresh, and the indoor temperature is generally between 18 and 20 degrees. Celsius, and the humidity is preferably between 60% and 65%.

(IV) Health Education

1. Stop tobacco and alcohol at least 4

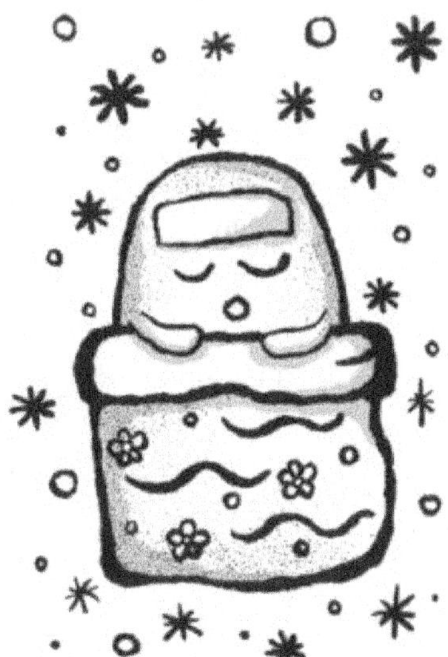

weeks before treatment. Prioritize warmth, rest, and avoid overexertion to minimize risks.

2. Drink plenty of water during radiotherapy.

3. For patients who have received chemotherapy, smoke for a long time, or have poor lung function, their condition should be closely monitored to detect and prevent the disease early, and patients should be guided to perform respiratory function exercises.

4. Family members should spend more time with patients and provide support in daily life. Care and psychological counseling are provided to enable patients to maintain a good mental state and build up confidence in overcoming the disease.

5. Pulmonary rehabilitation:

(1) Deep and slow breathing (pursed lip breathing), inhale through the nose and exhale through pursed lips, with the ratio of inhalation to exhalation time being 1: 2 or 1: 3. Try to inhale deeply and

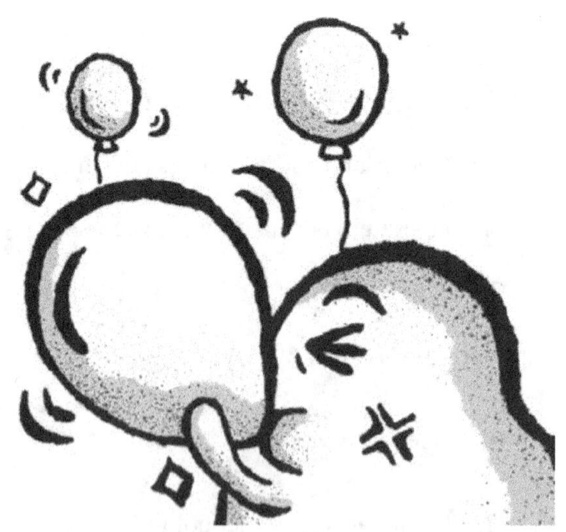

exhale slowly, 7 to 8 times per minute, twice a day, each time for 10 to 20 minutes.

(2) Physical exercise: (a) Stair climbing, the time is based on patients' tolerance, twice daily; (b) Alternate walking/jogging outdoors every morning and evening. Method: Walk for 50 minutes, jog for 50 minutes; (c) Do squats on the spot, start with 5 each time and gradually increase, 3 times/day. All exercises require nurse supervision.

(3) Diaphragmatic Breathing: Let the abdomen bulge when inhaling, and concave when exhaling, to develop a steady and slow abdominal breathing habit. Breathe deeply and slowly, and try to breathe via the nose instead of the mouth.

(4) Blowing balloons, bottles, and breathing function exercisers to strengthen deep breathing.

(5) Effective cough and sputum

A. Sit leaning forward with the neck slightly bent, master diaphragmatic breathing, and emphasize deep inhalation.

B. Place hands on patients' abdomen and exhale three times to feel the contraction of their abdominal muscles. Practice making the "K" sound to feel the tightening of patients' vocal cords, the closing of their glottis, and the contraction of their abdominal muscles.

C. Take a deep, relaxed breath, followed by a sharp double cough. Patients can apply appropriate pressure to patients' abdomen with their hands.

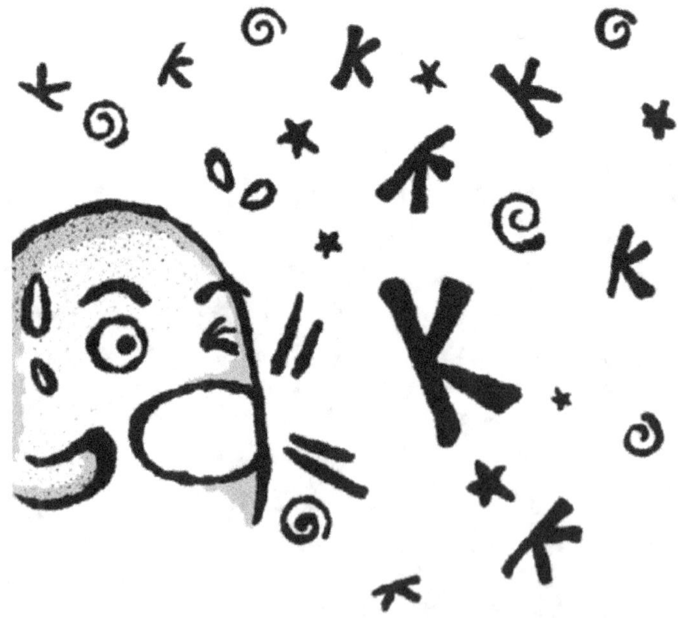

4. Radiation esophagitis

Radiation esophagitis occurs when normal esophageal mucosa within the irradiation field often becomes congested and edematous during radiotherapy for patients with malignant tumors in the chest and head and neck. This condition typically manifests as dysphagia, substernal burning, and localized pain worsening after eating. This is called radiation esophagitis.

(I) Clinical manifestations

Typical clinical manifestations include swallowing pain or retrosternal pain, which usually develops within 1 week or several weeks after radiotherapy and are often mild initially. In severe cases, there may involve excruciating chest pain, fever, choking, difficulty breathing, vomiting, hematemesis, etc. Be especially alert to the occurrence of esophageal perforation and esophageal fistula.

(II) Treatment

Clinical treatment principles: anti-inflammatory, protection of esophageal mucosal repair, pain control and nutritional support. Should symptoms become severe, radiotherapy may be temporarily suspended.

1. Symptomatic treatment

Provide high-calorie, high-protein, high-vitamin, easily digestible foods. Initiate partial or total parenteral nutrition if oral intake is compromised.

2. Medication

(1) Glucocorticoids: Such as dexamethasone, prednisone, and multivitamins to mitigate radiation damage.

(2) Digestive tract mucosal protective agents: Such as Smecta or Visco.

(3) Acid suppressants: Prevent gastric reflux irritation.

(4) H_2 receptor blockers: Such as ranitidine.

(5) Proton pump inhibitors: Such as omeprazole.

(6) Relieve esophageal smooth muscle spasm and protect esophageal mucosa.

(7) Anti-infection treatment.

(8) Enhance cellular immunity.

(9) Treatment with traditional Chinese medicine.

3. In addition to the above treatments, irradiation can be suspended or the interval between treatments can be extended if necessary.

(III) Nursing

1. Oral care management

Keep patients' mouth clean, pay attention to oral hygiene, rinse the mouth with warm salt water or antibacterial mouthwash. Brush the teeth every morning and evening, rinse the mouth or brush the teeth after meals to prevent bacteria from invading the esophageal mucosa and aggravating radiation esophagitis.

Choose suitable mouthwashes, such as normal saline or sodium bicarbonate solution. Encourage patients to rinse mouth frequently, especially after meals. Avoid using mouthwashes with alcohol content, which could irritate oral mucosa and cause mucosa dryness. Hold Kangfuxin solution orally to reduce inflammation and edema. Esophageal mucosal protectants can be used before radiotherapy. Patients can also consume 100g yogurt pre-radiotherapy whereby it forms a protective coating, mitigates radiation damage, repairs the damaged mucosa and prevents bacterial invasion. Concurrently, monitor vigilantly for strictures, ulcers, or perforation signs.

2. Dietary care

Instruct patients to consume liquid, semi-liquid or easy-to-swallow food, and encourage patients to eat more high-protein, high-vitamin, low-fat, and easily digestible food. The speed of eating should be slow. Oral tablets should be crushed to take to avoid lumps stuck in the narrow part of the esophagus and to reduce the chemical stimulation and physical damage of food to the mucosa. Eliminate tobacco, alcohol, sour food, overly salty, spicy and irritating food. Avoid crude fiber, hard, and fried items. Prevent bone-containing dishes from damaging the esophageal mucosa. Do not eat sticky food to avoid sticking to the surface of the esophagus and forming an obstruction. Drink a little warm water after meals to flush residues on the esophageal wall to reduce the inflammatory response of the esophagus. It is not advisable to lie flat after meals to avoid causing reflux of food digestive juices. Radiation inhibits saliva secretion, causing thirst and dry mouth. Encourage patients to hydrate with >2500mL warm water daily, which is conducive to the discharge of toxins.

3. Pain management

Observe the location, nature, degree and duration of patients' pain, and teach them ways to distract attention, such as self-relaxation, hypnosis, listening to music, etc. Take analgesics, antibacterial and anti-inflammatory, and digestive mucosal protection mixtures. Give painkillers as directed by doctors. For swallowing pain, utilize painkillers or appropriate amounts of local anesthetics in divided doses to treat the symptoms, such as 1% procaine, 2% lidocaine, etc. Educate patients to self-assess pain levels using standardized scales and emphasize immediate reporting of escalating symptoms to healthcare providers for prompt medication adjustment.

(VI) Health Education

As radiation esophagitis is a primary complication of thoracic radiotherapy, meticulous nursing care becomes critically important. Nurses should provide psychological care for patients during radiotherapy to make them fully prepared and eliminate their negative psychological state of nervousness, anxiety and fear.

5. Radiation proctitis

Radiation proctitis refers to rectal inflammation caused by the rectal mucosa being exposed to ionizing radiation or high doses of radiation that exceed the organ's tolerance dose.

(I) Clinical manifestations

Rectal bleeding is bright or dark red, and usually occurs during bowel movements. It is usually a small amount of bleeding, but occasionally severe.

After rupture, necrotic tissue will fall off and be discharged with a foul odor, and there will be soreness or burning pain in the anorectal area. Later, tenesmus will occur due to irritation of the sphincter.

Radiation proctitis is classified as acute and chronic.

1. Acute radiation proctitis

Refers to acute proctitis caused by the rectum (mainly mucosa) being exposed to ionizing radiation within half a year.

2. Chronic radiation proctitis

It is caused by the prolongation of acute radiation proctitis or direct irradiation for half a year, resulting in interstitial fibrosis, chronic rectal inflammation, intestinal stenosis, ulcers and fistula formation.

3. Complications

The main complications caused by radiation enteritis include intestinal stenosis and intestinal obstruction, rectovaginal fistula, rectovesical fistula or ileal and sigmoid colon fistula, gastrointestinal ulcers and perforation, and the induction of colon and rectal cancer.

4. Treatment

The treatment of radiation proctitis generally includes conservative treatment, such as anti-inflammatory hemostasis, retention enema, hyperbaric oxygen, etc.

5. Supportive care

Patients should rest in bed, eat soft, nutritious food with little residue, keep bowel movements smooth, take a hot water sitz bath after defecation, and apply hot compresses to the anus to reduce local irritation.

(II) Systemic therapy

1. Intestinal inflammation control

2. Traditional Chinese Medicine

The main purpose is to strengthen the body, nourish the blood and replenish Qi, while also clearing away heat and dampness to promote ulcer healing and subside inflammation.

(III) General management

During the acute phase, patients should rest in bed strictly and follow the diet principle of being non-irritating, easy to digest, rich in nutrition, and having multiple small meals. Fiber intake should be limited, and intravenous high-nutrient therapy can be used for patients with severe diarrhea.

Topical therapies include:

1. Medicated enemas. Smectite powder 3g in 80–100mL warm water, retained twice daily.

2. Surgical indications: Rectal stenosis, even obstruction, severe bleeding and fistula formation.

(IV) Nursing

1. During the acute phase, patients should rest in bed to reduce pain and fatigue, maintain smooth bowel movements, take a hot water sitz bath after defecation, and apply hot compresses to the anus to reduce local irritation. The nature of the abdominal pain should be observed. If the pain is obvious, indomethacin suppositories can be used.

2. Maintain anus and perineum clean, wear loose underwear, cleanse with warm water after bowel movements, and apply antibiotic ointment/petroleum jelly as needed.

3. Closely observe the shape, volume and nature of the stool. Antidiarrheal drugs can be used for those with obvious diarrhea. Avoid consuming raw or cold vegetables, fruits high in fiber, milk and dairy products.

4. Administer IV fluids when necessary to maintain fluid balance and prevent water and electrolyte imbalance caused by diarrhea.

5. Take antibiotics as prescribed by doctors and use retention enemas to control infection.

6. Psychological support: Prior to radiotherapy, patients should be informed of potential adverse reactions. Clinicians must establish a good relationship with patients, and enhance their sense of trust. When patients address frequent bowel movements and pain associated with radiation proctitis, clinicians should provide empathetic reassurance and clear explanations about these symptoms, enabling patients to understand both the treatment process and anticipated complications. This approach reinforces therapeutic confidence and promotes treatment adherence.

7. Diet care

(1) During the acute phase, patients should consume low-fat, bland, residue-free, and less irritating foods, while restricting dairy and lactose-containing products.

(2) Strengthen nutrition, consume high-calorie, high-protein food to compensate for the nutritional loss caused by long-term diarrhea. The supply can be gradually increased according to patients' digestion and absorption tolerance, prioritizing high-energy (40 kcal/kg/day) and high-protein (1.5 g/kg/day) diets with premium-quality proteins constituting 50%.

(3) Ensure adequate vitamins (such as vitamin C, E, E, A, and B group) and sufficient inorganic salts to compensate for the nutritional loss caused by diarrhea.

(4) Strictly limit fats and dietary fiber by avoiding eating foods that are high in irritants and fiber, such as spicy foods, sweet potatoes, radishes, celery, raw vegetables, fruits, as well as irritating onions, ginger, garlic, coarse grains, dry beans, etc.

(5) Implement small frequent meals to reduce the burden on the intestines.

(6) Eliminate sugar-rich foods, raw/cold dishes, and any substances causing gastrointestinal irritation.

(V) Health education

1. Before each radiotherapy session, evacuate bowels while maintaining a full bladder to minimize rectal radiation exposure.

2. Sustain regular bowel movements during radiotherapy to reduce the risk of constipation causing damage to the rectum and perianal skin and mucosa.

3. Instruct patients to consume small and frequent meals, provide adequate calories, and eat high-protein, high-vitamin, low-residue foods. Those with constipation can eat high-fiber foods. Those with abdominal pain and diarrhea can eat low-fat, high-protein foods which are low in residue and

easy to digest, consistently avoiding irritants.

4. Cultivate lifestyle habits including tobacco/alcohol/coffee cessation and abstinence from icy foods.

5. Establish structured routines ensuring adequate rest and sleep.

6. Participate in appropriate physical exercise to improve physical fitness and relax the mind.

6. Radiation cystitis

Radiation cystitis is congestion, edema and ulcer bleeding of the bladder mucosa caused by ionizing radiation.

(I) Clinical manifestations

The clinical manifestations of radiation cystitis can be divided into acute radiation cystitis and chronic cystitis. It starts with sudden, painless gross hematuria and is mainly manifested by persistent or recurrent, difficult to control gross hematuria, often accompanied by frequent urination and urgency. Some patients experience painful urination due to infection.

(II) Treatment

Common treatments for radiation cystitis include pharmacotherapy, hyperbaric oxygen, intravesical instillations, fulguration, and interventional procedures. For mild cases, symptomatic control with antibiotics and hemostatics to alleviate bladder irritation and bleeding.

Hyperbaric oxygen therapy. If mild radiation cystitis cannot be cured by conservative treatment, hyperbaric oxygen therapy can be added. Bladder instillation: Patients with moderate radiation cystitis can be treated with bladder instillation.

(III) Nursing

(1) For patients with severe radiation cystitis and recurrent macroscopic hematuria, administer intravesical medications per protocol after complete bladder emptying. Instruct patients to turn over frequently. This will enable the medication to fully come into contact with the inner wall of the bladder, achieving the effects of anti-inflammatory, hemostasis, promoting epithelial tissue repair and mucosal healing. For patients with severe bleeding, fresh blood should be transfused to correct anemia and improve overall condition.

(2) For mild-moderate acute radiation cystitis, conservative treatment is mainly used. Patients are advised to drink 1000-2000 mL of water every day Anti-infection, hemostatic and symptomatic treatments are used in a timely manner to relieve bladder irritation symptoms after each urination. Pay attention to cleaning the external genitalia and the urethral opening after each urination to prevent retrograde infection.

(3) Indwelling catheter care: During the indwelling catheterization, the purpose of catheterization should be explained to patients to alleviate their anxiety and fear. Patients should actively cooperate with the treatment, properly fix the catheter to avoid bending or folding, ensure that the urine

bag is lower than the bladder level, prevent retrograde infection, and keep the urethral opening clean. For patients with hematuria, the amount and color of hematuria, the presence of blood clots, should be observed and recorded. For patients with long-term indwelling catheterization, frequent catheter changes are not recommended, and bladder function exercises should be performed.

(4) Adjunctive pharmacotherapy: Implement prescribed anti-infectives/hemostatics as needed.

(5) Patients who have been bedridden for a long time should turn over frequently and observe the pressure on their skin to avoid the occurrence of pressure sores. Bed sheets should be arranged in a timely manner to avoid moisture and stimulation from excrement. Nutrition should be strengthened, lying positions should be changed frequently, and bony prominences should be protected.

(6) Basic care: Keep perineum clean, take good care of the skin for patients with vesicovaginal fistula, and keep bed clean, dry and free of contamination.

(7) Diet care: Eliminate spicy, irritating and gas-producing foods to reduce abdominal distension symptoms. Emphasize bland diet with > 2000mL daily hydration.

(IV) Health education

(1) Before pelvic radiotherapy, patients should be advised to empty their bladder. During intracavitary radiotherapy, gauze should be stuffed into the vagina to increase the

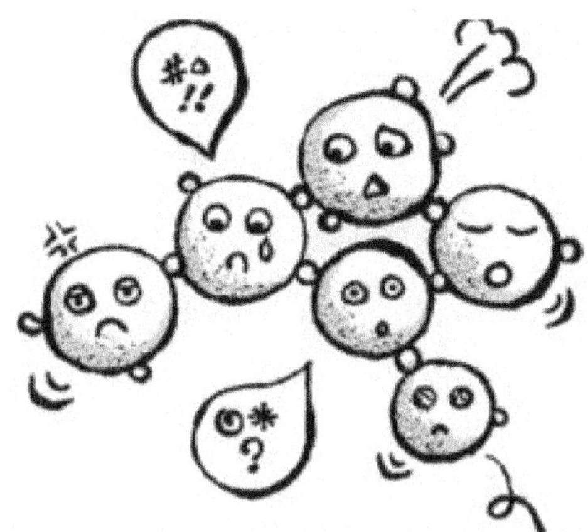

distance between the radiation source and the bladder and to reduce bladder involvement;

(2) Keep perineum cleanliness to prevent urinary tract infection;

(3) Avoid constrictive clothing.

(4) Abstain from tobacco/alcohol. Consume more fresh vegetables and diuretic fruits, etc., encourage drinking more water, more than 2000 mL of water per day, increase urine volume, and accelerate the excretion of toxins in the body.

(5) Maintain good living habits, increase activity appropriately according to physical condition, and ensure adequate rest and sleep;

(6) Develop good eating habits. Eat slowly, select soft, chewy, and digestible food.

(7) Schedule regular follow-ups, seek immediate care for symptom

changes.

7. Radiation-induced hematopoietic system reactions and Injuries

When the body undergoes radiation exposure, hematopoietic stem cells and immature blood cells rapidly decrease in number while their ability to multiply declines or ceases entirely. This leads to reduced levels of mature blood cells in the bloodstream.

I. Thrombocytopenia

(I) Clinical manifestations

(1) Bleeding may occur in the skin, gums, nose, vagina, gastrointestinal tract, or urinary system.

(2) When platelets drop below 20×10^9/L, it is easy to cause intracranial hemorrhage, manifested as headache, vomiting, and impaired consciousness.

(II) Nursing

(1) When platelet count drops below 50×10^9/L, patients should limit physical activity, prevent injuries and constipation, and avoid lifting heavy objects. Patients with severe thrombocytopenia should absolutely stay in bed and suspend activities.

(2) Keep systolic blood pressure under 18.7 kPa (140 mmHg) to prevent intracranial hemorrhage;

(3) Avoid NSAIDs (e.g., ibuprofen) and aspirin-containing medications;

(4) Avoid traumatic procedures such as intramuscular injections. Local pressure must be applied for more than 5 to 10 minutes after injection.

(5) Prevent all kinds of injuries and bleeding. Promptly detect bleeding in the skin and mucous membranes; use soft toothbrushes and do not brush the teeth too hard to prevent damage to the gums and mucous membranes and cause bleeding. Pay close attention to bowel movements and urination to promptly detect indications of gastrointestinal or urinary tract bleeding. Should bleeding occur, promptly administer hemostatic medications as prescribed to control the situation.

(6) Use specific cell growth factors (platelet growth factor, interleukin) and transfuse platelets;

(7) Dietary care: Provide high-protein, high-vitamin, easily digestible soft food, avoid hard, rough food, keep normal bowel movements, and avoid straining during defecation.

(III) Health education

(1) Keep warm and prevent colds;

(2) Physical activity must be minimized to avoid injuries, with strict bed rest implemented if necessary;

(3) Avoid actions that increase abdominal pressure and pay attention to laxatives and cough suppressants;

(4) Reduce the chance of mucosal damage: Eat soft food, avoid picking noses or ears, avoid using hard-bristled toothbrushes, or oral rinses instead.

II. Neutropenia

(I) Clinical manifestations

(1) Dizziness, soreness of limbs, decreased appetite, and fever;

(2) When white blood cell counts fall below 1.0×10^9/L, severe infections can rapidly develop in any organ system.

(II) Nursing

(1) Monitor body temperature closely to promptly detect signs of infection such as fever.

(2) For debilitated patients, deep breathing exercises are encouraged. For bedbound cases, perform regular repositioning and back percussion to prevent

(3) Minimize the risk of infection caused by exogenous microorganisms by avoiding contact with unhygienic fruits, vegetables and other plants, animals and their excrement, vaccinated people or patients with infectious diseases (such as chickenpox, herpes zoster, influenza and common cold, etc.).

(4) Patients should develop good hygiene habits, pay attention to food hygiene, oral rinsing after eating, and strengthen perineal cleaning after

urination and defecation.

(5) Protect skin/mucous membranes from injuries while ensuring proper wound care.

(6) Take a chest X-ray and check blood routine daily or alternate-day.

(7) Use broad-spectrum antibiotics empirically and change antibiotics based on the results of drug sensitivity tests.

(III) Health education

(1) Wash hands frequently;

(2) Avoid crowded places and contact with ill individuals.

(3) Never share food, cups, tableware or other daily necessities such as toothbrushes with others;

(4) Use soft toothbrushes to clean teeth and gums. If recommended by doctors or nurses, patients can use mouthwash to prevent oral ulcers.

III. Hemoglobin reduction

(I) Clinical manifestations

Pale skin, dull complexion, pale nails, palms, lip and eyelid mucosa, dizziness, tinnitus, memory loss, inattention, and in severe cases, low fever.

(II) Nursing

(1) Pay attention to rest and do moderate activities. For those with severe

anemia, the rest method, activity intensity and duration of each activity should be determined according to the degree of decline in their activity tolerance.

(2) Use specific cell growth factors (erythropoietin) and red blood cell transfusion

(3) Advise patients to eat more foods that are good for blood circulation, such as red dates, peanuts, etc.

(4) Diet care: A reasonable diet, including high-fiber and fresh fruits and vegetables, balanced nutrition, including essential nutrients such as protein, sugar, fat, trace elements and dietary fiber. A combination of meat and vegetables, and a variety of food.

(III) Prevention

The most important preventive measure for radiation-induced bone marrow suppression is to monitor blood counts regularly, at least once a week.

8. Radiation-induced heart disease

Radiation-induced heart disease refers to a group of clinical and pathological conditions involving damage to the heart caused by radiation exposure during radiation therapy for adjacent tumors. This condition specifically describes myocardial lesions that develop following exposure to radioactive materials.

(I) Nursing

(1) Maintain bed rest with oxygen administration and emotional stability; adopt a comfortable lying position according to the condition;

(2) Provide high-calorie, high-protein, high-vitamin, easily digestible semi-liquid or soft foods, and limit sodium intake;

(3) Observe chest and precordial pain, pay attention to the nature of the pain, apply ice packs locally and minimize coughing or position changes to alleviate pain. For dry fibrinous pericarditis, lie on the left side to relieve pain.

(4) Closely observe changes in breathing, blood pressure, pulse, heart rate, complexion, etc. If cardiac tamponade symptoms appear, such as pale complexion, rapid breathing, irritability, cyanosis, decreased blood pressure, irritating dry cough, tachycardia, and distended jugular veins, immediately notify the physician for rescue;

(5) For high fever: timely cooling down, promptly changing patients' clothes, regularly measuring and recording body temperature, ensure warmth to prevent chilling and respiratory infections.

(6) Provide explanations, comfort, and psychological care.

(II) Health education

(1) Maintain a healthy diet by increasing intake of fruits, vegetables,

beans, and nuts, abstain from alcohol and tobacco.

(2) Engage in regular physical activity with exercise tailored to individual capacity.

(3) Ensuring adequate sleep.

9.Radiation-induced brain injury

Radiation brain injury refers to changes in normal brain tissue function and morphology caused by ionizing radiation treatment of head and neck tumors, intracranial tumors, cerebrovascular malformations and other diseases, or accidental exposure to ionizing radiation to the brain.

(I) Clinical manifestations

Radiation-induced brain injury can be classified into three phases based on the timing of symptom onset: acute phase, early delayed reaction phase, and late delayed reaction phase.

1. Acute phase

Presents with altered mental status and consciousness, including headache, nausea, vomiting, intracranial hypertension and impaired consciousness. These symptoms are generally considered reversible.

2. Early delayed reaction

Occurs 1 to 6 months after radiotherapy. Patients may experience increased excitability, loss of appetite, dizziness, drowsiness, learning and memory impairment, irritability, fatigue, and even exacerbation of tumor-related symptoms and signs. Most of the above symptoms and signs are recoverable.

3. Late delayed reactions

This stage is irreversible damage. It occurs 6 months to several years after irradiation. Localized radiation necrosis manifests as changes in movement, sensation, language, and receptive ability, epilepsy, and increased intracranial pressure.

(II) Nursing

Closely monitor changes in the patient's condition.

(1) Headache, dizziness, and slurred speech are the main symptoms of radiation-induced brain injury. Closely observe headache severity, vital signs, consciousness, pupil changes, and be alert to the occurrence of brain herniation. Secondly, provide a quiet and comfortable sleeping environment to ensure adequate sleep, maintain emotional stability, and avoid the stimulation of negative emotions.

(2) During vomiting, maintain airway patency to prevent aspiration and ensure oral hygiene.

(3) For patients with limb weakness or unsteady gait, they should take preventive measures to prevent falls.

(4) For patients with high fever, cerebral hypoxia and cerebral edema may be aggravated. Apply effective cooling measures while monitoring skin color during cooling to prevent frostbite.

(5) Strengthen respiratory care. Promptly and thoroughly clear airway secretions to maintain respiratory patency.

Part 16: Radiotherapy Emergency and Nursing

Radiotherapy emergencies refer to emergent radiotherapy administered as the primary treatment for oncologic emergencies, encompassing three clinical scenarios: conditions requiring immediate radiotherapy (within 24 hours) to relieve critical compression caused by tumor enlargement or infiltration, including central nervous system/spinal cord compression, superior vena cava syndrome, and airway obstruction at the trachea or its bifurcation; second, emergencies that occur during radiotherapy, such as high fever, coma, nasal and nasopharyngeal bleeding, hemoptysis, and laryngeal dyspnea, require urgent treatment; third, tumor patients with other internal and external emergencies such as angina pectoris, gastric perforation, acute appendicitis, lobar pneumonia, etc, require emergency management.

1. Superior vena cava syndrome

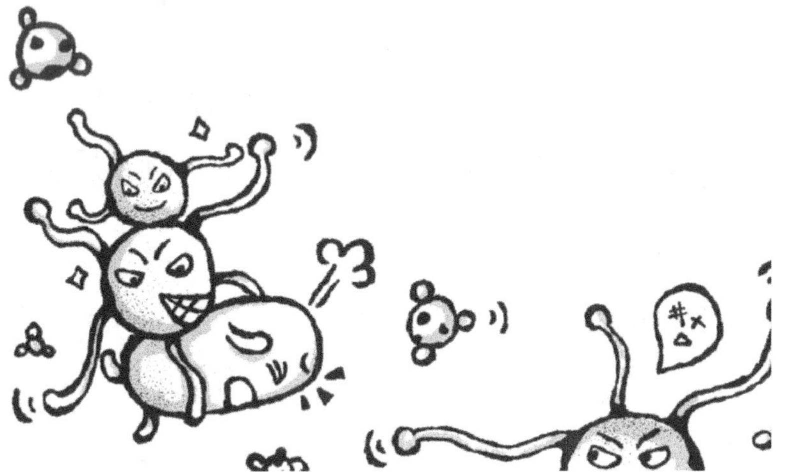

Superior vena cava syndrome, also known as superior vena cava obstruction syndrome, is a group of clinical syndromes characterized by congestion and edema of the face, neck and upper limbs, and varicose veins of the upper body. It represents a relatively common emergency in oncology.

(I) Symptoms and signs

(1) Symptoms: dyspnea, facial swelling, cough, hoarseness, wheezing, headache, blurred vision, swollen tongue, nasal congestion, dizziness, nausea, etc.;

(2) Physical signs: Physical examination may reveal distended neck

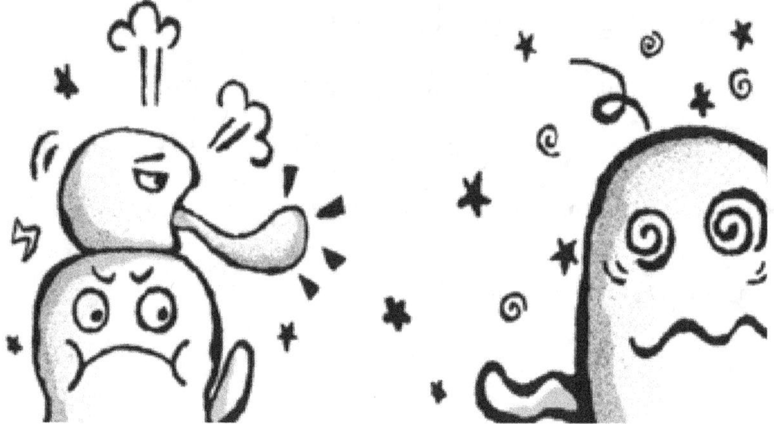

veins, congestion of the face and upper body, swelling of the upper limbs, cyanosis, abnormal mental state, drowsiness, lethargy and coma, optic disc edema, conjunctival edema, syncope, etc.

(II) Nursing

1. Condition monitoring

Closely observe facial, neck, and upper limb edema severity, and monitor for the symptoms of dyspnea, hypoxia, increased intracranial pressure, or altered consciousness.

2. Positioning care

Place the patient in semi-Fowler's, high Fowler's, or high-pillow position with the head elevated 30-45°. This facilitates blood return to the head and neck, lowers the diaphragm, expands the chest cavity, increases lung ventilation, and relieves breathing difficulties. Simultaneously, keep lower limbs dependent to reduce venous return.

3. Airway management

Administer continuous low-flow oxygen via nasal cannula. If severe coughing, shortness of breath, and cyanosis of the lips, high-flow mask oxygen inhalation should be given immediately to correct the symptoms of hypoxia.

4. Selection of intravenous infusion site

Strictly limit the amount of fluid replacement and control the infusion speed. Do not puncture and infuse fluid in the upper limb vein, external jugular vein, and subclavian vein to avoid increasing the blood volume of the superior vena cava and aggravating the compression symptoms.

5. Pressure injury prevention

Use pressure-relieving mattresses or water cushions under the hips. Cover the pressure-prone areas with Mepilex (soft polysilicone) dressings, and closely monitor skin integrity.

6. Blood pressure measurement

Measure BP on the left upper arm; perform bilateral comparison if needed. Because the superior vena cava reflux is obstructed, it increases the pressure of the right brachial artery and the blood pressure of the right upper limb. Therefore, it is not appropriate to use the right upper limb to measure blood pressure.

7. Limit sodium and water intake

Limit dietary sodium intake and fluid consumption to maintain fluid balance. Accurately record 24-hour intake and output, and observe changes in body weight.

8. Chemotoxicity monitoring

During intravenous chemotherapy, avoid lower extremity veins, especially for blistering agents or highly irritating drugs. Central venous catheters are recommended. For high-dose chemotherapy, igorously monitor blood routine, electrolytes, liver and kidney function, etc.

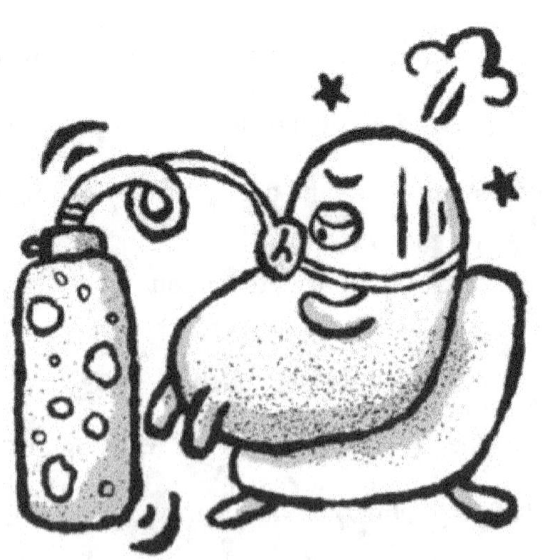

9. Radiation reaction

observation

Observe for symptoms of radiation pneumonitis such as fever, shortness of breath, cough, chest pain, and dyspnea. Monitor for symptoms of radiation esophagitis such as pain behind the sternum, nausea and vomiting, and worsening swallowing obstruction after eating.

10. Psychological support

Provide counseling for patients and families to encourage treatment adherence and mitigate negative emotions.

(III) Health education

1. Psychological counseling

Superior vena cava compression syndrome has an acute onset, obvious clinical symptoms, and forced posture, which can easily lead to negative emotions in patients. Nurses should provide empathetic support, monitor emotional changes, actively listen, identify concerns promptly, and offer psychological guidance. Guide patients to use relaxation techniques, and explain previous successful cases to increase their confidence in

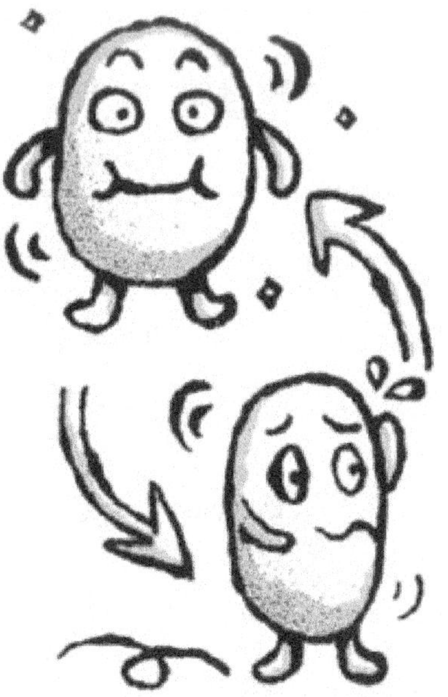

overcoming the disease.

2. Dietary guidance

Emphasize nutritional importance. Provide a high-protein, high-vitamin, high-sugar, low-salt, low-fat, easily digestible diet, limit the sodium salt and water intake in food. Recommend small, frequent meals. For radiation esophagitis: patients should be guided to eat light, easily digestible, warm and cool liquid or semi-liquid, and avoid spicy, coarse, hard, hot and other irritating foods. The eating speed should not be too fast, chew slowly, rinse the mouth after eating, and take 50-100 mL of warm salt water orally to flush the esophagus, reducing food residues in the lesion, and reducing local inflammation and edema. For severe odynophagia: Swish 15–20 mL of a pre-meal mixture (250 mL 0.9% saline + 10 mg lidocaine + 50 mL vitamin B_{12} + 10 mg dexamethasone) to alleviate pain and facilitate eating.

3. Promote expectoration

Instruct patients to effectively cough, expectorate and back percussion to prevent respiratory tract infections. Assist patients to change their positions regularly. Provide infusion guidance and explain the necessity of lower extremity intravenous infusion to improve patient compliance.

4. Posture guidance

Guide and assist patients to assume the correct body position, and explain the importance of taking semi-Fowler's or high-Fowler's posture with dependent lower limbs, emphasizing its hemodynamic benefits.

5. Activities and functional exercise

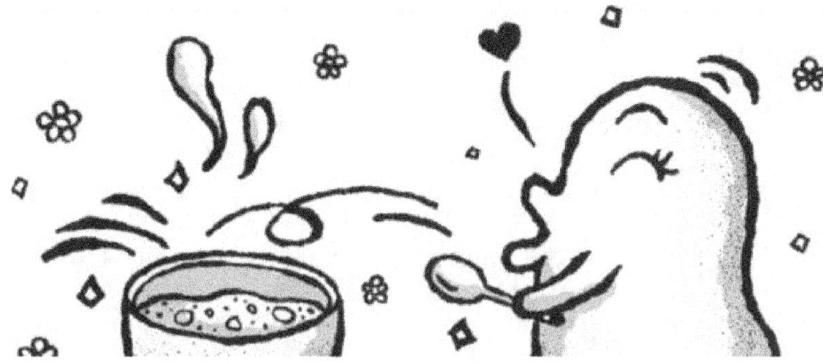

Patients should minimize activities and avoid fatigue. They can move limbs in bed appropriately and get out of bed as soon as possible after their condition improves to avoid the formation of blood clots. For radiation pneumonitis: Guide through breathing exercises (pursed-lip breathing, chest expansion).

6. Skin care

Instruct patients on self-care of radiation-field skin, keep clean and dry, change underwear frequently, and wear loose, sweat-absorbent, cotton clothes. Iodine, ethanol, medicated oil, and adhesive tape are prohibited on radiation-field skin. The water temperature should be appropriate when bathing. Soap, shower gel, etc., are prohibited. Not to wipe off the radiotherapy marks on their bodies. Cut nails frequently and prevent scratching. Triethanolamine cream (Biafine) can be applied topically to radiation-field skin 3 times a day. Instruct patients to take measures to protect edematous skin and prevent pressure sores.

7. Regular check-ups and follow-up if any discomfort occurs.

2. Spinal cord compression

Spinal cord compression is a common clinical syndrome caused by primary or metastatic tumors compressing the spinal cord, leading to pathological changes such as edema, degeneration, and necrosis, ultimately leading to loss of spinal cord function. It represents one of the most serious complications in tumor patients.

(I) Symptoms and signs

Early relief of spinal cord compression is very important for preserving neurological function and quality of life. Therefore, vigilance for signs of compression is essential. The proportion of neurological function recovery in patients with delayed diagnosis is only 15%.

The first symptom of spinal cord compression is typically back pain, which is localized or radiating, or a combination of both. The pain worsens with coughing, activity, lying flat, and back muscle tension. As the condition progresses, sensory deficits, muscle weakness, sphincter dysfunction, and ultimately paralysis may develop rapidly.

(II) Nursing

1. Condition monitoring

Early diagnosis is crucial for the treatment of spinal cord compression.

Closely monitor patients' status, promptly assess muscle strength, pain level, skin compression, sensory nerve dysfunction, excretion disorders, vital signs, and psychological status. The prodromal symptoms of spinal cord compression should be discovered as early as possible. If there are any abnormalities, report to doctors in time and assist in treatment.

2. Pain management

Assist patients to take a comfortable position and closely observe adverse drug reactions such as constipation, nausea and vomiting, dizziness, itching, respiratory depression, motor and cognitive dysfunction, etc.

3. Urinary dysfunction care

Instruct patients to maintain fluid intake at ~2000mL/day. Keep catheter patency, observe urine color, volume, and characteristics. Keep the perineum dry and clean, with twice-daily cleansing. If the urine is turbid, flush the bladder with 0.1% furazolidone solution twice a day. Bladder dysfunction caused by spinal cord injury should be trained, and the catheter should be clamped during the day and opened every 2 hours or when there is an urge to urinate.

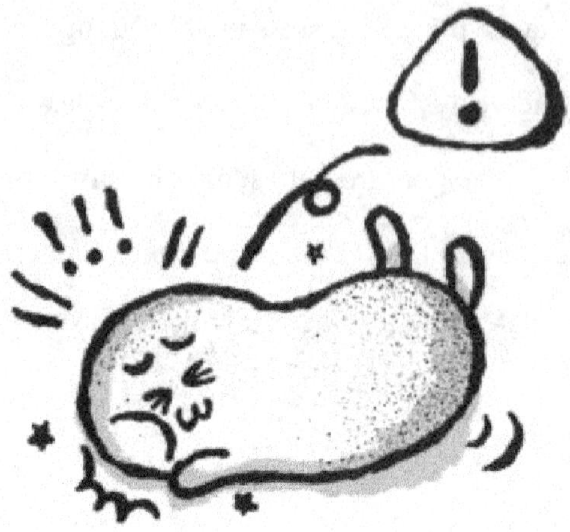

4. Fall prevention

Patients with decreased limb strength should be alert to the occurrence of falls. Promptly assess the risk of falls, and set up fall warning signs. Ensure the safety of the surrounding environment, with bright lights, no obstacles, dry floors, and handrails in wards, toilets, and corridors. Place daily necessities that patients often use within easy reach.

Use bed guards according to patients' conditions and arrange nursing care reasonably.

5. Pressure injury prevention

Use anti-pressure sore beds or air mattress. Reposition every 2 hours to improve circulation. Perform log-rolling with head-neck-trunk alignment to prevent spinal injury. When turning over, move gently, avoid pulling, pushing, and dragging. Protect the skin over the bone prominence and cover it with Mepilex foam dressing or a transparent dressing. Apply Saifurun on the skin under local pressure to relieve the local blood supply disorder caused by skin pressure.

6. Thrombosis prophylaxis

To prevent thrombosis in long-term bedridden patients, they should strengthen limb function exercises and activities. Observe both lower limbs

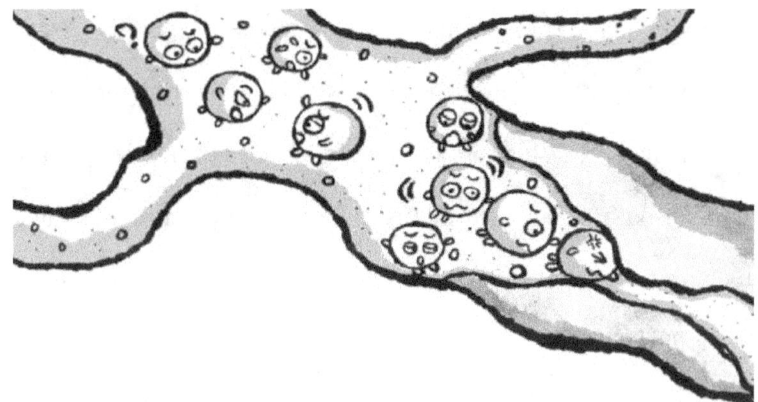

swelling, measure leg circumference regularly, avoid lower-extremity IV access, and apply elastic stockings or bandages in the early stage.

7. Limb function exercise

Assist or guide patients to perform functional exercises to prevent limb contracture, deformity and muscle atrophy. These mainly include massage, maintaining the functional position of the affected limb, active and passive movement, sit-up exercise, etc. When to start active and passive limb exercises depends largely on spinal stability. It is generally believed that patients could start doing exercise when pain is within a tolerable range or after treatment. Patients with unstable gait should be alert to falls when they are moving.

8. Hypostatic pneumonia prevention

Encourage fluid intake and coached coughing (with back percussion/abdominal pressure). Strengthen nutrition, keep warm, and prevent upper respiratory tract infections. Guide patients to perform respiratory function exercises and check lung function regularly. Strengthen exercise. For example, bedridden patients should perform limb function exercises, or sit by the bed or wheelchair to reduce muscle atrophy and weakness caused by long-term bed rest. Reposition every 2–4 hours. For thick sputum, undergo nebulization inhalation or oral expectorants, etc. If accompanied by dysphagia, nasogastric feeding should be given in time to avoid aspiration or choking, which may lead to or aggravate aspiration pneumonia.

9. Sensory deficit care

Patients require 24-hour round-the-clock care. Close observation should be conducted to check for any redness, swelling, pallor or other abnormalities in the patient's limb skin. Strictly prohibit hot water bottles or ice packs to prevent burns and frostbite. Close monitoring should also be carried out to detect any symptoms of radiating osteomyelitis such as numbness, crawling sensation, stabbing pain or aching sensation in the limbs.

10. Psychological support

Explain treatment methods to patients and their families, provide psychological support, avoid negative emotions, encourage patients to actively cooperate with treatment, and jointly participate in the formulation and implementation of nursing plans.

(III) Health education

1. Psychological counseling

Demonstrate understanding and compassion. Encourage patients to adopt a positive outlook on their illness. Share recovery success stories to help strengthen their confidence in overcoming the disease.

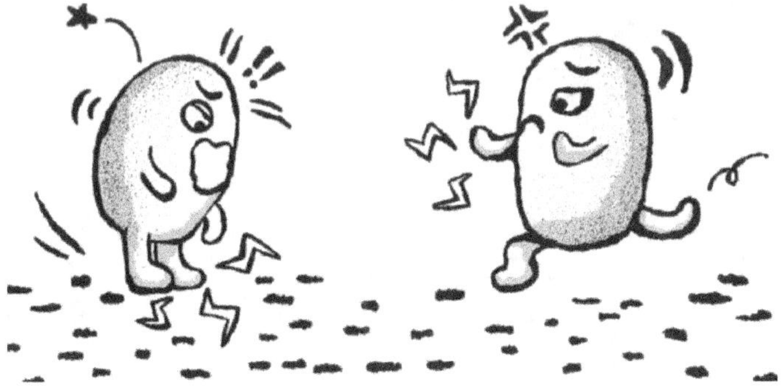

2. Dietary guidance

Strengthen nutrition to enhance the body's resistance. Provide high-protein, high-vitamin, high-fiber, easily digestible foods, including chicken, lean meat, eggs, fish, beans, milk, sweet potatoes, carrots, fungus, bananas, watermelons, apples, etc. Encourage adequate fluid intake.

3. Medication guidance

Educate patients and families on cancer pain management principles and medication protocols. Instruct patients to take medication on time and not to reduce or stop medication without authorization. Teach patients and their families pain assessment tools, and inform them of adverse drug reactions and medication precautions. Advise patients to consume easily digestible, low-fat, and crude fiber-rich diets, and ensure a daily water intake of 2000-3000 mL. Exercise appropriately if the condition permits, which helps to reduce or prevent gastrointestinal reactions. For dizziness, change positions slowly, sit on the bed for 3 minutes first, then stand by the bed for 3 minutes.

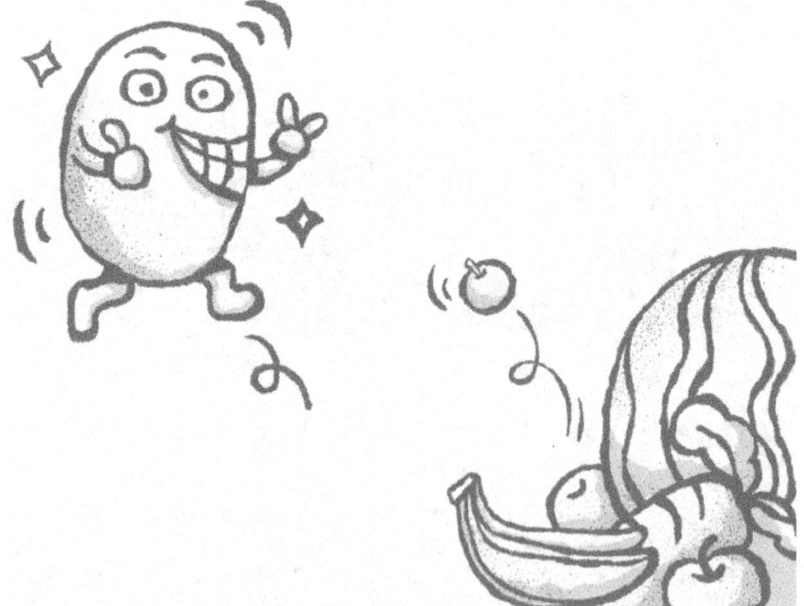

Family members should support them during activities to avoid falls or falling out of bed.

4. Skin care

Instruct patients on self-care of radiation-field skin, keep clean and dry, change underwear frequently, and wear loose, sweat-absorbent, cotton clothes. Iodine, ethanol, medicated oil, and adhesive tape are prohibited on radiation-field skin. The water temperature should be appropriate when bathing. Soap, shower gel,

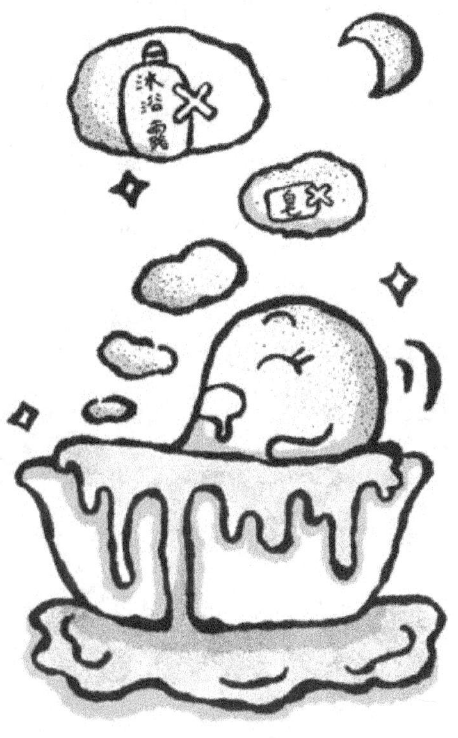

etc., are prohibited. Not to wipe off the radiotherapy marks on their bodies. Cut nails frequently and prevent scratching. Triethanolamine cream (Biafine) can be applied topically to radiation-field skin 3 times a day. Concurrently educate patients and families on the mechanism and importance of pressure injury prevention, teaching preventive methods to avoid ulcer development.

5. Safety precautions

Be careful to prevent falls. Instruct patients to wear non-slip shoes when getting out of bed or moving around. Put on or take off clothes, socks, and shoes while seated. Guide patients that they can only ambulate with nurse/family assistance and move slowly. Do not attempt the activity if experiencing dizziness, headache, or discomfort.

6. Activities and functional exercise

Instruct patients and their family in joint mobility and muscle training while maintaining physiological curvature of spine. During repositioning, use the log-rolling technique (head-neck-trunk alignment) to prevent spinal torsion and cord injury. Instruct and assist patients to do appropriate limb exercises, such as flexion and extension of the knee, elbow, and toe joint, raising the lower limbs, and massaging the muscles to promote blood circulation and to prevent muscle atrophy and limb function degeneration. Keep the foot in a functional position and place a pillow under the sole.

7. Regular check-ups and follow-up if any discomfort occurs.

3. Intracranial hypertension

Intracranial hypertension is a syndrome in which the volume of cranial cavity contents increases or decreases due to intracranial diseases, exceeding the compensatory capacity of the cranial cavity, resulting in intracranial pressure persistently higher than 200 mmH$_2$O, with headache, vomiting and optic disc edema as the main clinical manifestations.

(I) Symptoms and signs

1. Symptoms

Most patients experience headaches. Severe headaches may be accompanied by nausea and projectile vomiting, which is unrelated to food intake. A headache may temporarily subside after vomiting. When combined with tumor bleeding, it is often misdiagnosed as a cerebrovascular accident. Depending on the location of brain metastasis, patients may also exhibit mental confusion, impaired consciousness, diplopia, blackouts, dizziness, epilepsy, etc.

2. Physical signs

Papilledema is a key diagnostic indicator. In addition, different signs may appear depending on the location of brain tissue compression: restricted eye movement, decreased vision, hemiplegia, aphasia, lateral sensory disturbance, etc. Patients with diffuse meningeal metastasis or tumor-induced subarachnoid hemorrhage present with meningeal signs.

(II) Nursing

1. Posture guidance

Instruct patients to stay quiet and rest in bed, and raise the head of the bed 15 to 30 degrees to facilitate intracranial venous return and reduce cerebral edema. Comatose patients should be placed in lateral positioning to promote respiratory secretion clearance.

2. Condition monitoring

Closely observe changes in consciousness, pupils, and vital signs.

Monitor for worsening original symptoms. Immediately notify the physician and initiate interventions if signs of acute increased ICP develop.

3. Airway management

Clear respiratory secretions promptly, give oxygen continuously or intermittently to alleviate cerebral edema, and reduce intracranial pressure. Patients with impaired consciousness and difficulty expectorating should cooperate with doctors to perform tracheotomy as soon as possible. Turn patients over and press their backs regularly to prevent lung complications.

4. ICP monitoring

Dynamically track ICP changes to prevent abrupt elevation triggering herniation. Patients should pay attention to keeping the pipeline unobstructed, recording intracranial pressure, maintaining the airtightness of the drainage or monitoring system, and preventing retrograde infection.

5. Fever control

Reduce fever in hyperthermic patients to improve cerebral oxygenation.

6. Safety precautions

Control seizures promptly. Avoid emotional excitement, severe coughing, constipation, etc. Prevent and control epileptic seizures to avoid aggravating cerebral hypoxia and cerebral edema, and prevent patients from falling out of bed, suffocation and other accidents.

7. Fluid restriction

The daily fluid replacement volume should not exceed 2000 mL, the urine volume should be maintained at no less than 600 mL per day, and the 24-hour intake and output should be recorded.

8. Adverse reactions after taking medicine

Observe response to dehydrating agents and closely monitor electrolyte status to prevent the occurrence of hyponatremia, hypokalemia, acute heart failure, and pulmonary edema.

9. Bowel management

Avoid straining during defecation. For constipation, administer laxatives or low-pressure enemas with minimal fluid volume.

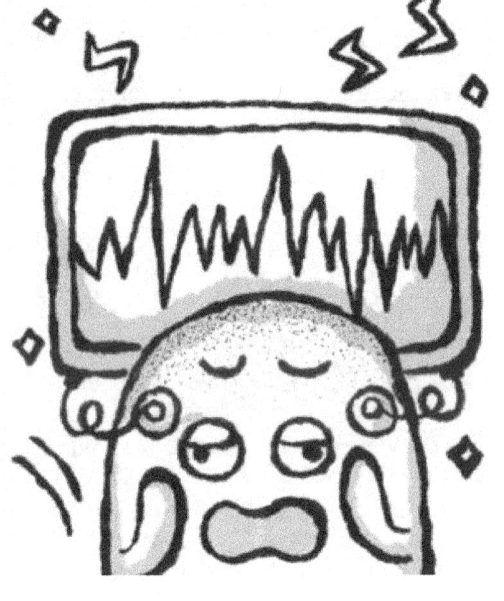

10. For patients scheduled for surgery: Complete all preoperative preparations systematically.

11. Ventricular drainage care

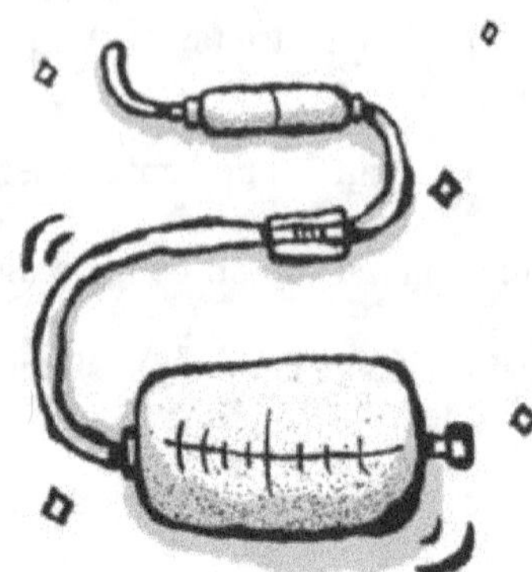

(1) The drainage tube should be properly fixed and maintained unobstructed. The opening of the drainage tube should be 10 to 15 cm above the level of the lateral ventricle. Clamp the tube temporarily during patient repositioning or drainage bag replacement to prevent air entry or CSF reflux that may cause intracranial infection.

(2) Observe and record the color, volume and properties of cerebrospinal fluid. Adjust the height of the drainage tube according to the drainage volume, and control the drainage speed and volume.

(3) Catheter removal protocol: The drainage tube is usually placed for 3 to 4 days, at which time the brain edema has subsided and the intracranial pressure has decreased. It should not exceed 5-7 days to avoid intracranial infection due to prolonged time. Perform a head CT scan before tube removal, and try to raise the drainage bag or clamp the drainage tube for 24 hours to assess cerebrospinal fluid (CSF) circulation patency. When removing the tube, clamp the catheter first to prevent CSF backflow and infection risk. After tube removal, apply a pressure dressing at the insertion site. Instruct the patient to maintain strict bed rest with minimized head movement. Closely observe the puncture site for bleeding or CSF leakage. Monitor for altered

consciousness, pupillary changes, aphasia or limb convulsions, etc. Report any abnormalities to the physician immediately.

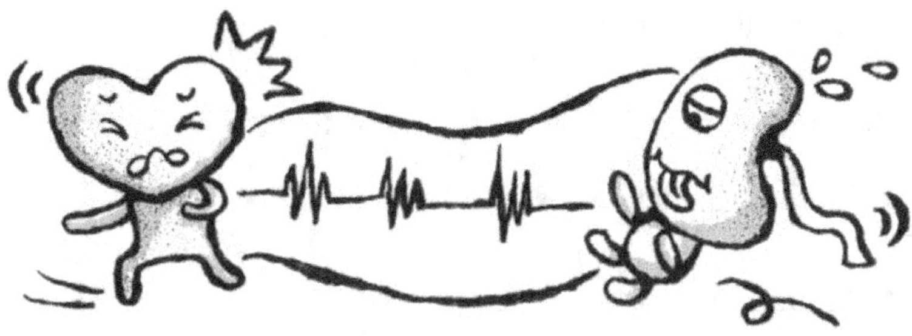

(III) Health education

1. Dietary guidance

Consume primarily soft, easily digestible foods that are high-calorie, high-protein, vitamin-rich, and fiber-rich. Avoid dry or hard foods.

2. Psychological support

Maintain a calm mindset and stable emotions. Avoid emotional agitation and shouting, as these may increase intracranial pressure.

3. Behavioral guidance

Instruct patients to avoid coughing, constipation, lifting heavy objects, etc., to prevent a sudden increase in intracranial pressure from inducing brain herniation.

4. Symptom vigilance

Seek immediate medical attention if experiencing a progressive headache with vomiting unresponsive to routine treatment. Attend scheduled follow-ups.

5. Airway management

During vomiting: The head should be tilted to one side to prevent vomitus from blocking the airway and causing suffocation.

6. Posture guidance

Rest in bed with the head of the bed elevated 15°~30 to facilitate intracranial venous return and reduce cerebral edema.

7. Functional Exercise

Keep the indoor environment quiet and encourage patients with neurological sequelae to actively engage in functional exercises.

4. Acute tumor lysis syndrome

Acute tumor lysis syndrome (ATLS) is the most urgent complication in the process of tumor treatment, characterized by rapid lysis of tumor cells induced by anticancer treatment. This results in life-threatening cardiac arrhythmias or acute renal failure, constituting a critical clinical syndrome.

(I) Clinical manifestations

Mild cases may not cause any obvious discomfort. Clinical symptoms depend on the severity of metabolic abnormalities:

(1) Acute presentation: Typically presents with high fever (39–40°C);

(2) Hyperuricemia: Nausea, vomiting, drowsiness, hematuria, increased uric acid, renal insufficiency, and occasional gout attacks;

(3) Hyperkalemia: Fatigue, muscle aches, arrhythmias, may progress to cardiac arrest;

(4) Hyperphosphatemia & hypocalcemia: Neuromuscular hyperexcitability, carpopedal spasm, skin itching, ocular and joint inflammation, and renal impairment;

(5) Metabolic acidosis: Fatigue, tachypnea, and severe cases: nausea, vomiting, drowsiness, and coma;

(6) Azotemia & renal insufficiency: Oliguria, anuria, rapid increase in blood creatinine and urea nitrogen.

(II) Nursing

1.Dietary management

Reduce exogenous intake of potassium, phosphorus, and purine. During the nursing process, educate patients and their family not to eat lean meat, bananas, orange juice and other potassium-rich foods. Cut the vegetables with high potassium content into pieces and cook them in water, then discard the water to reduce the potassium content. Implement strict low-phosphorus (less than 600 mg of phosphorus per day) and low-purine diets. Strictly limit purine-rich foods like fish, shrimp, animal brains, offal, seafood, chicken, duck and shellfish.

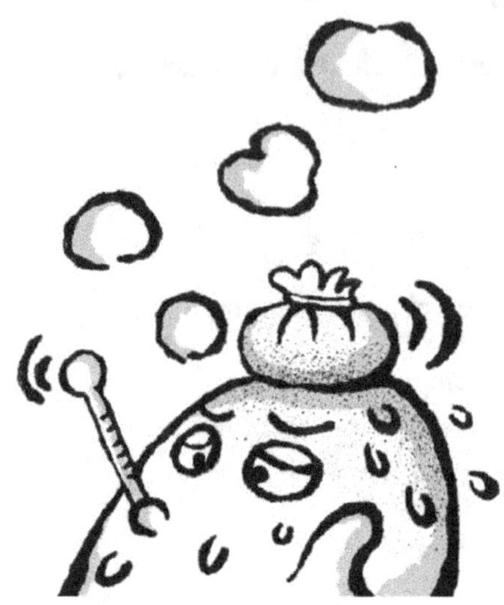

2. Pressure injury prevention

Accurately assess the risk of pressure sores and closely observe the pressure on the skin. Use pressure-relieving mattresses and reposition every 2 hours to enhance circulation. Be gentle when turning patients over and avoid pulling, pushing, or tugging. Protect the skin over bony prominences and cover with Mepilex foam dressings or transparent dressings. Apply Sanyrene® lotion to compressed skin to alleviate microcirculatory compromise.

3. Radiation reaction observation

Observe for symptoms of radiation pneumonitis such as fever, shortness of breath, cough, chest pain, and dyspnea. Monitor for symptoms of radiation esophagitis such as retrosternal pain, nausea, vomiting, and worsening swallowing obstruction after eating.

4. Symptomatic care

(1) Hyperkalemia diet management: Avoid eating foods high in potassium, such as dark vegetables, bananas, kelp, etc.

(2) Hyperphosphatemia diet management: Hyperphosphatemia results from inorganic phosphate released by lysed tumor cells depositing in the kidneys, impairing renal function and further reducing urinary potassium/phosphate excretion. Therefore, patients should avoid eating foods high in phosphorus, such as milk.

(3) Hypocalcemia management: Manifestations include muscle cramps, arrhythmias, altered consciousness, etc. Patients are prone to movement, and have numbness and tingling sensations around the mouth and fingertips. Increase calcium-rich foods (e.g., milk, eggs). For chronic supplementation: administer oral calcium and vitamin D_3.

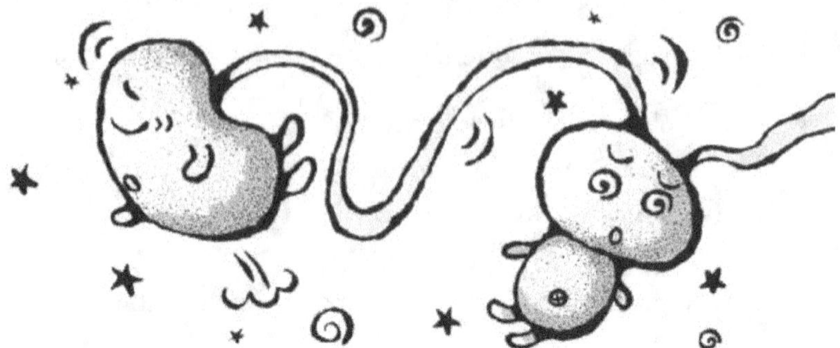

(4) Hyperuricemia care: Urate released by the lysis of a large number of tumor cells is deposited in the kidneys, causing renal impairment. Urate deposited in the joints can cause gout. Urea/creatinine elevations occur due to renal precipitation of urates/phosphates.

(i) Urine Output Monitoring: Urine output should be observed during radiotherapy and chemotherapy, and a sudden decrease in urine output should be considered a complication.

(ii) Dietary Control: Strengthen dietary guidance and implement low-purine diet. Encourage fluid intake >2000mL/day to maintain high urine output.

5. Comfortable care

Instruct patients to maintain bed rest. Keep the ward clean, tidy and quiet. Promote emotional calmness. If clinically permitted, engage in appropriate weight-bearing activities to prevent excessive calcium loss. Ensure safety during activities to prevent injury.

(III) Health education

1. Psychological support

Understand and care about patients and encourage them to treat the disease correctly. Share recovery success stories to strengthen confidence in overcoming the disease.

2. Dietary guidance

Strengthen nutrition to boost immunity while reducing the intake of exogenous potassium, phosphorus, and purine. Consume foods with low-potassium, low-phosphorus (less than 600 mg of phosphorus per day) and low-purine diet. Strictly limit purine-rich foods, such as fish, shrimp, animal brains, offal, seafood, chicken, duck, and shellfish. Patients are encouraged to drink more water to facilitate the excretion of uric acid sediment.

3. Skin care

Instruct patients on self-care of radiation-field skin, keep clean and dry, change underwear frequently, and wear loose, sweat-absorbent, cotton clothes. Iodine, ethanol, medicated oil, and adhesive tape are prohibited on radiation-field skin. The water temperature should be appropriate when bathing. Soap, shower gel, etc., are prohibited. Not to wipe off the radiotherapy marks on their bodies. Cut nails frequently and prevent scratching. Triethanolamine cream (Biafine) can be applied topically to radiation-field skin 3 times a day. Concurrently educate patients and families on the mechanism and importance of pressure injury prevention, teaching preventive methods to avoid ulcer development.

4. Safety precautions

Be careful to prevent falls. Instruct patients to wear non-slip shoes when getting out of bed or moving around. Put on or take off clothes, socks, and shoes while seated. Guide patients that they can only ambulate with nurse/family assistance and move slowly. Do not attempt the activity if experiencing dizziness, headache, or discomfort.

5. Regular check-ups and follow-up if any discomfort occurs.

5. Hypercalcemia

Hypercalcemia refers to an abnormally elevated serum ionized calcium concentration. It is the most common metabolic complication of cancer, with an incidence of 15% to 20%. According to statistics, individuals with breast cancer, multiple myeloma, and non-small cell lung cancer most frequently develop hypercalcemia.

(I) Clinical manifestations

Symptoms are manifested in the digestive, motor, nervous, urinary, and circulatory systems. When the disease lasts for a long time, calcium deposits may occur in tissues, such as conjunctival and periarticular deposits and kidney stones. The clinical manifestations of hypercalcemia are related to the magnitude and speed of blood calcium increase.

1. Gastrointestinal symptoms

Early symptoms include anorexia, nausea, vomiting, and abdominal pain. They are often insidious and diagnostically challenging. In the late stage, constipation may occur, and in severe cases, paralytic ileus may occur. Calcium can stimulate the secretion of gastrin and gastric acid, increasing peptic ulcer risk. Calcium deposition in the pancreatic ducts can stimulate the secretion of large amounts of pancreatic enzymes, causing acute pancreatitis.

2. Neuropsychiatric symptoms

In the early stage, symptoms include fatigue, lethargy, apathy, drowsiness and depression. In the late stage, symptoms may include headache, muscle weakness, decreased tendon reflexes, irritability, unsteady gait, speech disorders, hearing, visual/auditory deficits, stupor, abnormal behavior, etc. In the case of hypercalcemic crisis, delirium, convulsions and coma may occur.

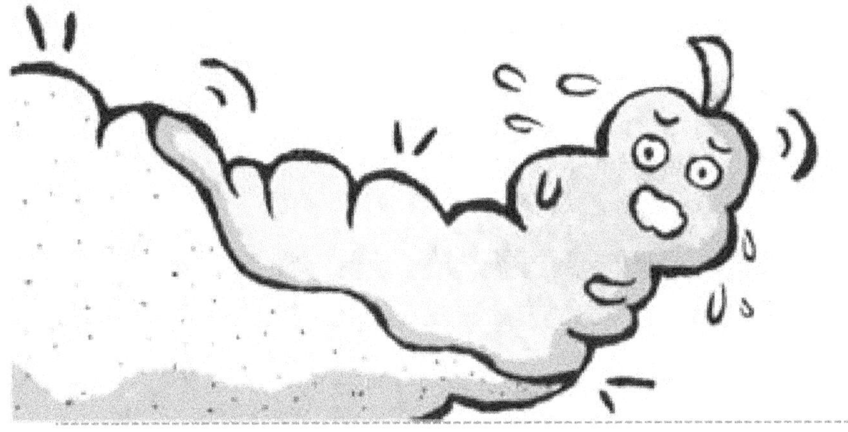

3. Renal symptoms

In the early stage, it may manifest as polyuria, polydipsia, and polydipsia. Calcium deposits in the renal parenchyma, causing interstitial nephritis, salt-losing nephropathy, and nephrocalcinosis, eventually developing into renal failure. It is also prone to urinary tract infections and stones.

4. Cardiovascular symptoms

Bradycardia and various arrhythmias often occur.

5. Respiratory symptoms

It can easily lead to lung infection, breathing difficulties, and even respiratory failure.

(II) Nursing

1. Condition monitoring

Observe changes in the patient's consciousness, vital signs, tendon reflexes, muscle tension, etc. Pay attention to exacerbation of pre-existing symptoms.

2. Psychological support

According to patients' personality, education level, personal background, and psychological needs, targeted communication should be conducted to help them cooperate with clinical treatment in a good mental state and build confidence in overcoming the disease. For patients with risk factors or early manifestations, explain hypercalcemia's symptoms, signs, and treatment plan to patients/families. Prepare them psychologically to prevent negative emotional responses.

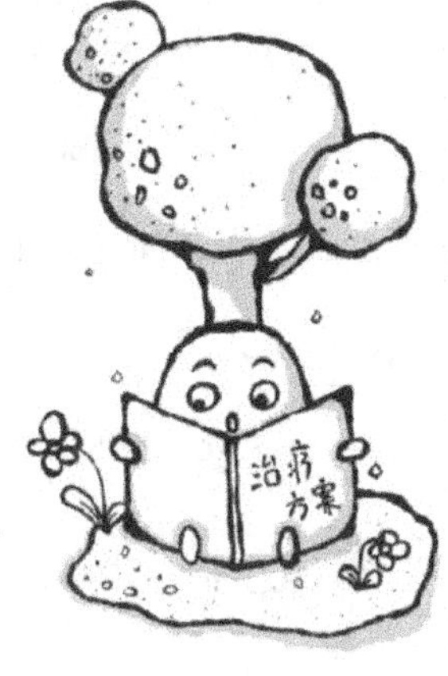

3. Diet management

According to patients' preferences, cooperate with nutritionists to appropriately improve the dietary patterns, meal timing, and food choices to ensure nutrition while preventing or mitigating hypercalcemia.

4. Medication management

Administer prescribed volume expansion to dilute serum calcium and enhance urinary calcium excretion. If necessary, use antiemetics, analgesics, antiarrhythmics, diuretics and blood calcium-lowering drugs. Monitor for adverse reactions.

5. Comfortable care

Instruct the patient to keep bed rest, reduce activities, and ensure adequate sleep, thereby effectively alleviating the physical symptoms. Maintain a clean, quiet environment and emotional calmness. Do appropriate activities when the condition allows, and ensure safety during activities to prevent injuries. For debilitated or unconscious patients: provide passive range-of-motion exercises.

6. Pressure injury prevention

Reposition every 2 hours to enhance circulation. Be gentle when turning patients over and avoid pulling, pushing, or tugging. Protect the skin over bony prominences and cover with Mepilex foam dressings or transparent dressings. Apply Sanyrene® lotion to compressed skin to alleviate microcirculatory compromise.

7. Radiation toxicity monitoring

Observe for symptoms of radiation pneumonitis such as fever, shortness of breath, cough, chest pain, and dyspnea. Monitor for symptoms of radiation esophagitis such as retrosternal pain, nausea, vomiting, and worsening swallowing obstruction after eating.

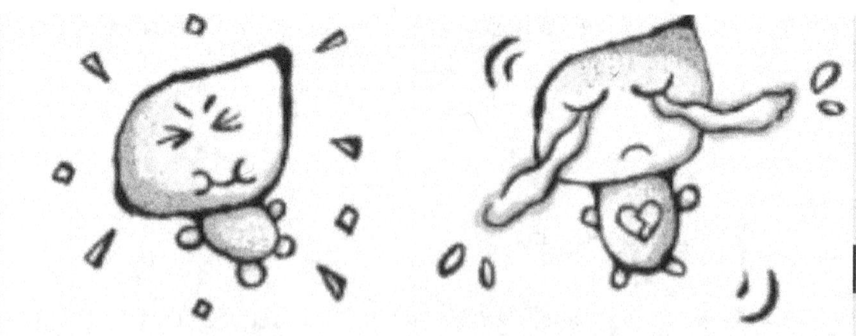

8. Airway management

Clear respiratory secretions promptly, give oxygen continuously or intermittently to alleviate symptoms such as fatigue, chest tightness, and dyspnea. Patients with impaired consciousness and difficulty expectorating should cooperate with doctors to perform tracheotomy as soon as possible. Turn patients over and press their backs regularly to prevent lung complications.

(III) Health education

1. Psychological support

To establish a good nurse-patient relationship, medical staff should understand and care about patients and encourage them to treat the disease correctly. Share recovery success stories to strengthen confidence in overcoming the disease.

2. Dietary guidance

Optimize nutrition to boost immunity while reducing the intake of high-calcium foods. Encourage >3000mL/day fluid intake to promote calciuresis, correct electrolyte imbalances, and improve acid-base balance.

3. Skin care

Instruct patients on self-care of radiation-field skin, keep clean and dry, change underwear frequently, and wear loose, sweat-absorbent, cotton

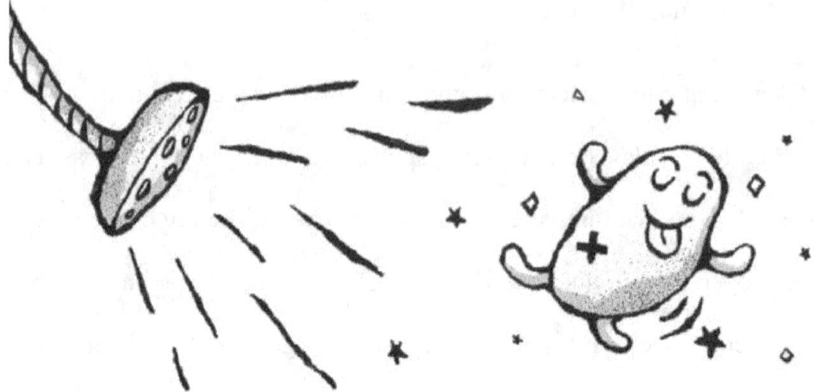

clothes. Iodine, ethanol, medicated oil, adhesive tape are prohibited on radiation-field skin. The water temperature should be appropriate when bathing. Soap, shower gel, etc., are prohibited. Not to wipe off the radiotherapy marks on their bodies. Cut nails frequently and prevent scratching. Triethanolamine cream (Biafine) can be applied topically to radiation-field skin 3 times a day. Concurrently educate patients and families on the mechanism and importance of pressure injury prevention, teaching preventive methods to avoid ulcer development.

4. Safety precautions

Be careful to prevent falls. Instruct patients to wear non-slip shoes when getting out of bed or moving around. Put on or take off clothes, socks, and shoes while seated. Guide patients that they can only ambulate with nurse/family assistance and move slowly. Do not attempt the activity if experiencing dizziness, headache, or discomfort.

5. Functional exercise

Encourage safe, supervised activity as tolerated by the patient's condition to prevent injury. For debilitated patients or those with impaired consciousness, provide assisted passive range-of-motion exercises.

6. Schedule regular follow-ups and seek immediate care for new symptoms.

6. Nasopharyngeal carcinoma (NPC) hemorrhage

Nasopharyngeal carcinoma is a malignant tumor originating from the roof and lateral walls of the nasopharynx. It is a malignant tumor with a special geographical and ethnic distribution worldwide and is one of the most common malignant tumors in China, accounting for the highest incidence among otorhinolaryngological cancers.

(I) Clinical manifestations

1. Bleeding may occur without warning, with blood suddenly flowing or gushing out of the nose or mouth.

2. Hemorrhage severity and symptoms

(1) When the amount of bleeding is small, there are generally no systemic symptoms.

(2) When the amount of bleeding is >500 mL, there may be early symptoms of shock such as pale complexion, cold hands and feet, irritability, mental tension, and increased heart rate.

(3) When the amount of bleeding is >1000 mL, symptoms such as apathy, slow reaction, cyanosis of the lips and extremities, cold sweat, decreased blood pressure, and oliguria may occur.

(II) Nursing

1. Condition Monitoring

Upon detecting a massive hemorrhage, nurses should remain calm, quickly identify the bleeding source and volume, assess the patient's status, notify doctors immediately, reassure the patient, and stabilize their emotions.

2. Posture guidance

Assist patients into a sitting, semi-sitting or or lateral position on the affected side. This is beneficial for the drainage of oral secretions. At the same time, it can lower the diaphragm, improve breathing conditions, and cushion airflow stimulation to the nasal passages, thereby reducing bleeding. If the bleeding is severe and the amount of bleeding is large, maintain patients in a head-down lateral position and avoid moving them unnecessarily. If necessary, apply pressure to the bilateral external carotid arteries.

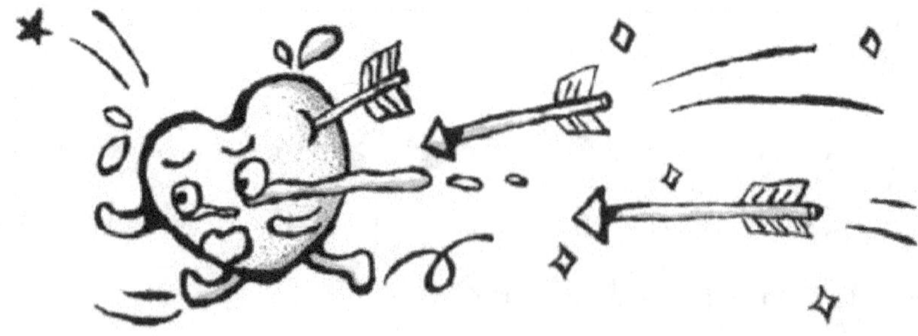

3. Airway management

Clear the airway immediately. Maintaining a patent airway is critical for successful resuscitation. Instruct patients not to swallow blood and administer high-flow oxygen therapy.

4. Volume expansion and hemostasis therapy

Rapidly establish at least two intravenous channels to quickly expand blood volume. Follow doctors' instructions to infuse low-molecular-weight dextran, whole blood, plasma, etc., to maintain effective circulation. Concurrently, administer hemostatic agents to prevent the onset of hemorrhagic shock.

5. Packing and hemostasis

Assist the physicians in using Vaseline gauze, posterior nasal packing or air bag rapid nasal packing to perform hemostasis. Once the bleeding is localized and symptoms subside, send patients to undergo nasal endoscopy as ordered to identify the bleeding site for cauterization.

6. Sedation therapy

Use sedative treatments such as diazepam or phenobarbital as directed by doctors.

7. Psychological support

Epistaxis is usually an emergency. Patients often feel nervous and fearful. Comfort patients, encourage them to stay calm, and help divert their attention to avoid heightened emotional tension, which will aggravate the bleeding. Address the concerns of both the patient and their family, encouraging active cooperation with treatment.

If the amount exceeds 500-1000 mL, the infusion must be accelerated. If the systolic blood pressure is <80 mmHg, the pulse is >120 times/minute, and shock occurs, it indicates that the blood loss is more than 1500mL. This mandates pressurized infusion of fluids and blood products.

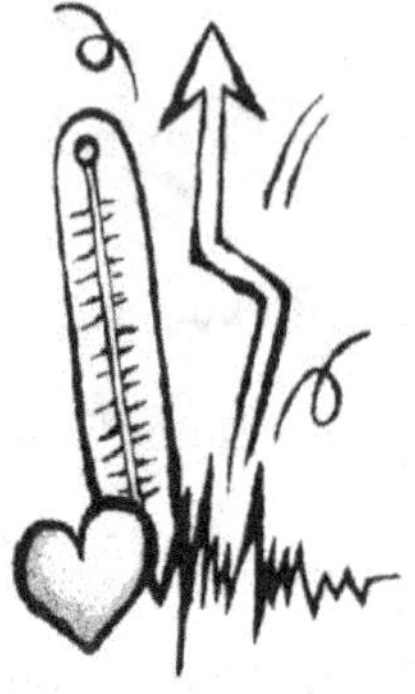

(III) Health education

1. Psychological support

Explain to both patients and their family that extreme anxiety and agitation can cause muscle tension in the throat and vasoconstriction, making bleeding control more difficult while also elevating blood pressure and worsening the bleeding. Care for and comfort patients, and guide them to take deep breaths. Sharing examples of previous successful cases can boost the patient's confidence in overcoming the condition and secure their full cooperation. At the same time, clean the blood stains on patients' clothes and bed sheets in time to relieve their tension.

2. Ensuring adequate rest

Strict bed rest with no physical activity is mandatory during active bleeding. Once the bleeding has completely subsided, patients can take a walk indoors according to their condition but must avoid strenuous activities. Patients can take a semi-sitting position and apply a cold towel or ice cubes to the forehead or both sides of the neck.

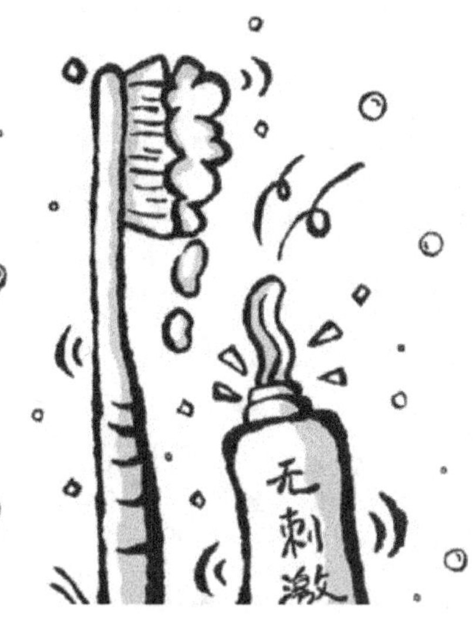

3. Maintain airway patency

Clear the respiratory tract, give oxygen inhalation, and instruct patients on how to breathe through the mouth to keep breathing smoothly. Crucially, advise patients not to swallow blood from the mouth. Instead, it should be spit into a designated container to allow observation of the blood's nature, color, and volume. Guide or assist patients with oral rinsing using solutions such as cetylpyridinium chloride gargle, Koutai gargle, and normal saline to eliminate oral odors and maintain hygiene. Keep the mouth and lips moist and cover them with moist gauze.

4. Medication guidance

Instruct patients to use 0.25% chloramphenicol ophthalmic solution or ofloxacin eye drops 4 times daily.

5. Nasal care

(1) Advise patients not to blow the nose, strenuous activities, violent coughing, sneezing, and forceful bowel movements, etc., as these actions may dislodge nasal packing, increase intravascular pressure, and trigger rebleeding.

(2) Patients should be warned not to remove the string of the posterior nasal plug without authorization, and pay attention to whether it is loose. Use ephedrine nasal drops several times daily to moisten the nasal cavity and packing materials, preventing discomfort from drying.

(3) The packing should be removed after 48 to 72 hours. Since the blood vessels in the damaged area have not yet been completely repaired, it is forbidden to blow or pick the nose. The blood clots left in the nasal cavity cannot be cleared by themselves to avoid rupture of blood vessels and bleeding again.

6. Dietary guidance

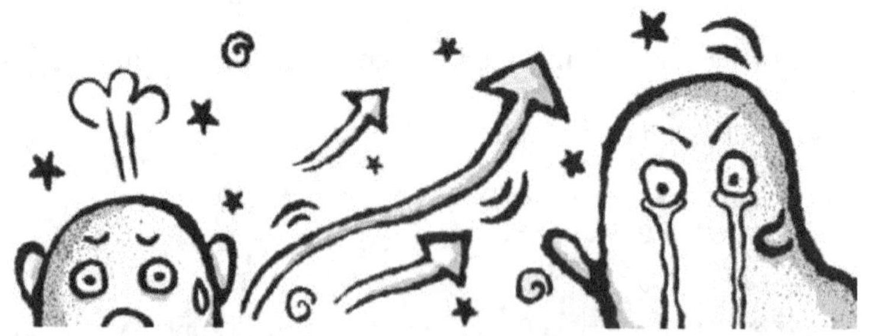

Patients with reduced or stopped bleeding should consume a warm, liquid, low-residue diet. Those with significant bleeding who underwent nasal packing should initially fast; after packing removal, transition to lukewarm/cool liquid or semi-liquid diets to minimize rebleeding risk before gradually advancing to regular diets. Crucially, avoid overheated, hard, spicy and stimulating foods. All meals should be eaten slowly to prevent choking or aspiration.

7. Hemoptysis

Hemoptysis refers to the process of bleeding from the respiratory organs below the larynx (i.e., trachea, bronchi, or lung tissue), which is expelled through the mouth via coughing. It is a critical and severe disease that threatens patients' lives. Notably, hemoptysis may arise not only from respiratory diseases but also from circulatory diseases, trauma, and other systemic diseases or systemic factors.

(I) Clinical manifestations

Recurrent hemoptysis may persist for several years or even decades, ranging in severity from blood-streaked sputum to massive bleeding. The volume of blood loss varies according to etiology and pathology, though it does not strictly correlate with disease severity. Minimal presentations include blood-tinged sputum, while severe cases involve sudden expulsion of hundreds or even thousands of milliliters of blood.

(1) Most patients with severe hemoptysis may have prodromal

symptoms such as chest tightness, an itchy throat, and a cough. The blood is typically bright red and frothy, often mixed with sputum. However, some patients do not have any prodromal symptoms and suddenly develop severe hemoptysis.

(2) When coughing up blood, symptoms such as chest tightness, difficulty breathing, cyanosis of the lips and nails, irritability, and pale complexion may suddenly appear. These are signs of suffocation and the condition is critical.

(3) Repeated massive hemoptysis, with cold limbs, profuse sweating, low hemoglobin, continuous drop in blood pressure, and even shock, are manifestations of circulatory failure. It is a critical deterioration.

(II) Nursing

1. Maintaining airway patency

Postural drainage and keeping the airway open are critical to successfully rescuing patients with massive hemoptysis. To minimize bleeding and prevent blood from entering unaffected lung areas, position the patient laterally on the affected side with the head turned to facilitate blood expulsion from the airway. Concurrently, clear oral blood and clots to prevent asphyxia. Should any of these critical choking signs emerge during bleeding:

(i) Sudden cessation of hemoptysis, with chest tightness and mental tension;

(ii) Patients are restless and urgently need to sit up to breathe;

(iii) Noise in the pharynx, sudden rapid breathing, and clenched teeth;

(iv) Interrupted projectile bleeding followed by dyspnea. Or patients open their mouths and eyes in amazement after a small amount of blood is ejected from the mouth and nasal cavity;

(v) In case of respiratory arrest, cyanosis, grasping hands, confusion, incontinence, etc., immediately place the patient in a head-down and foot-up position, firmly pat the back to expel tracheal blood by gravity. Use a mouth gag to open the oral cavity or tongue forceps to pull the tongue forward. Use a suction tube to suck with negative pressure to avoid blood clots blocking the airway and causing suffocation. Prepare for emergency endotracheal intubation or tracheostomy if required to evacuate obstructing clots.

2. Psychological support

Provide reassurance to both the patient and family members. Observe changes in patients' emotions, actively listen to concerns, and promptly address emerging issues. Deliver targeted psychological guidance, coaching the patient in relaxation techniques to alleviate fear and strengthen confidence in overcoming the condition.

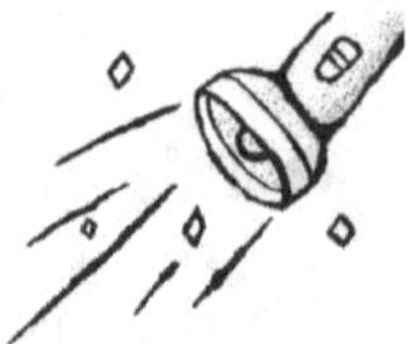

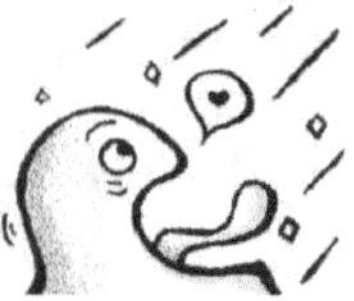

3. Oxygen therapy

Administer high-flow oxygen inhalation, control the oxygen flow rate at 6-8 L/min, and use an artificial respirator to assist breathing if necessary. Prepare rescue supplies such as tongue depressor, mouth gags, tongue forceps, suction device, simple artificial air bag, tracheotomy kit, etc. at the bedside.

4. Cough management

Patients with a cough can be given nebulized inhalation as prescribed by doctors to dilute the sputum. If accompanied by a severe cough, codeine can be taken orally.

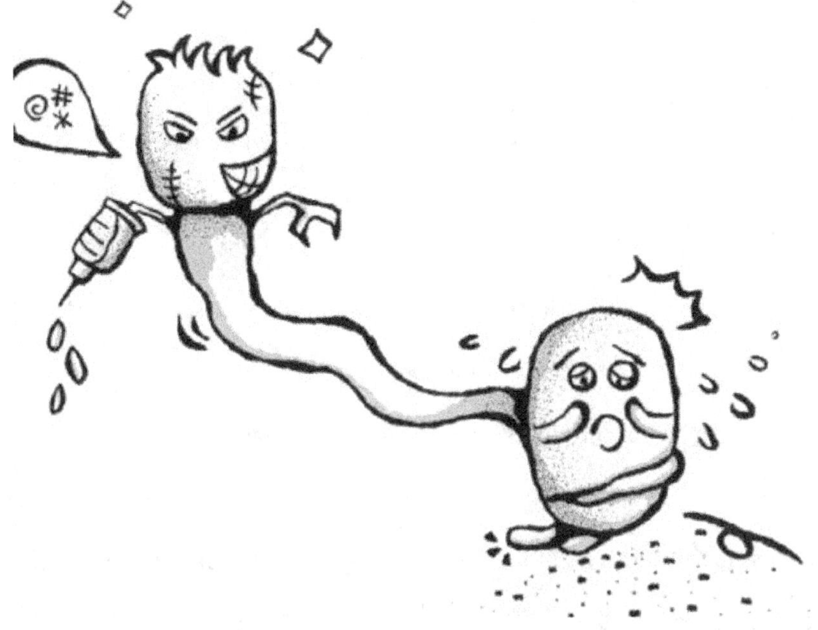

5. Ensuring adequate rest

Strengthen basic nursing care, keep the ward clean, bright and quiet. Absolute bed rest is mandatory after massive hemoptysis, with all non-essential movement strictly avoided to promote recovery.

(III) Health education

1. Psychological care

Since massive hemoptysis occurs suddenly and violently, patients often react with tension, fear, pessimism, and despair. Nurses should provide compassionate reassurance and demonstrate understanding. Coach patients in relaxation techniques to stabilize emotions and obtain their full cooperation. Instruct patients to cough up blood from the oropharynx as much as possible and not to hold their breath to prevent laryngeal spasm and blood discharge obstruction leading to suffocation. Clean blood from patients' clothes and bed units in a timely manner to relieve their tension.

2. Bed rest

Patients require strict bed rest for at least one week after bleeding cessation, with minimal repositioning. Assist patients to lie on the affected side and reduce the activity of the affected side to facilitate ventilation of the healthy side. Once clinically stable, patients may begin indoor walking but must avoid strenuous activities, severe coughing, and straining to defecate to prevent bleeding again.

3. Dietary guidance

Patients with severe hemoptysis require temporary fasting and intravenous nutritional support. Patients with minor hemoptysis or those whose hemoptysis has stopped should consume small amounts of warm and cool liquid food, with increased water intake. Avoid drinking strong tea, coffee, alcohol, hard, spicy and other irritating foods. After hemoptysis stops, patients can eat high-protein, high-calorie, low-fat, vitamin-rich and easily digestible liquid or semi-liquid food.

4. Maintaining bowel regularity

Educate patients on the critical importance of preventing constipation. Instruct them to eat foods such as bananas, dragon fruit, and carrots to keep bowel movements open. For existing constipation, administer glycerol enemas to facilitate bowel movements, preventing straining-induced increases in thoracic/abdominal pressure that may trigger or worsen bleeding.

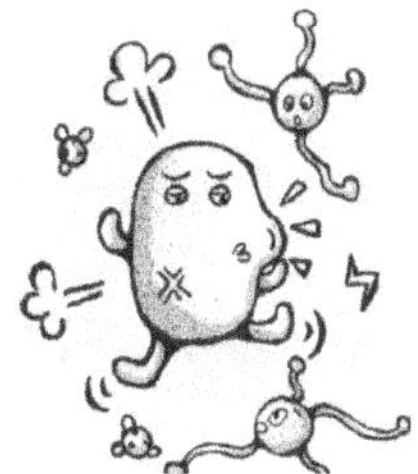

5. Oral hygiene

After hemoptysis episodes, instruct or assist patients to rinse their mouths to remove bad breath and increase comfort.

6. Prevent upper respiratory tract infections

Advise patients to keep warm, avoid catching colds, strengthen nutrition, ensure adequate sleep, and avoid respiratory tract infections.

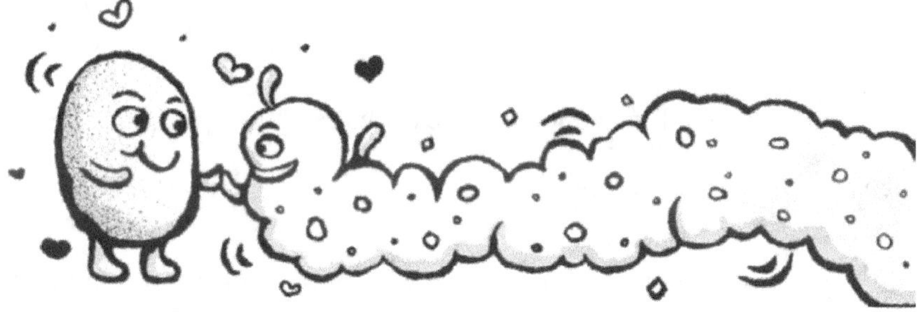

7. Post-Stability Rehabilitation Guidance

Do not overwork, and avoid severe coughing. Exercise appropriately, proceed step by step, and avoid strenuous exercise.

8. Disease knowledge education

Train patients and their family to recognize early warning signs, such as sudden agitation, cyanosis, dyspnea and other discomforts, immediately lie prone at a 45 angle with the head low and the feet high, pat the back gently to expel blood clots from the respiratory tract and oropharynx, and stay quiet to reduce the risk of suffocation due to massive hemoptysis.

8. Airway obstruction

Airway obstruction refers to ventilation obstruction caused by intrinsic or extrinsic pathologies of the respiratory tract.

(I) Clinical manifestations

Primary manifestations include dyspnea, wheezing and/or eating obstruction. Dyspnea severity is divided into 4 degrees:

Grade I: No dyspnea at rest, but inhalation dyspnea occurs during activity.

Grade II: Mild inhalation dyspnea occurs when at rest, aggravated by activity, without irritability.

Grade III: Obvious dyspnea, with visible retractions at the suprasternal fossa, supraclavicular fossa, intercostal space (triple retraction sign), as well as nasal flaring, sweating, irritability and mild cyanosis.

Grade IV: Symptoms are more severe, including cyanosis, pale complexion, and finally coma, asphyxiation leading to respiratory and cardiac arrest.

(II) Nursing

1. Condition monitoring

(1) Closely observe patients' consciousness, respiratory rate and rhythm, blood oxygen saturation, and lip and nail bed color to determine dyspnea severity grade. Administer moderate-flow oxygen therapy throughout.

(2) Functional training: Guide patients in changing their posture and breathing techniques to improve respiratory status.

(i) A commonly used posture to improve respiratory symptoms is to lean forward and use a table to support the arms and upper body to improve the function of the auxiliary muscles and increase ventilation capacity.

(ii) Breathing techniques include diaphragmatic breathing and pursed lip breathing. Diaphragmatic breathing involves relaxing shoulders, while placing hands on the lower edge of the ribs in the abdomen, inhaling through the nose, and holding breath by bulging patients' abdomen outwards against their hands. When exhaling, gently apply pressure under the ribs with your hands, and exhale slowly through the mouth. Meanwhile, pursed lip breathing requires nasal inhalation followed by exhalation through tightly pursed lips (as if whistling) with the chest leaning forward, maintaining an inhalation-to-exhalation ratio of 1:2 or 1:3 at a controlled rate of 7–8 breaths per minute.

2. Comfort management

Keep the environment clean and quiet, reduce adverse stimulation. For restless patients, administer sedatives as medically prescribed.

3. Psychological intervention

Patients with tumor-induced respiratory compression often experience intense fear, feelings of impending doom, or depressive symptoms. It is important to identify these psychological reactions and implement timely supportive interventions.

4. Postoperative care

Patients who undergo tracheotomy should be observed and cared for after the operation. After the operation, take a semi-sitting position, maintain airway patency while encouraging patients to cough up sputum. Perform suctioning using negative pressure as needed to clear oral/tracheal tube secretions, thereby preventing pulmonary infections. Instill 0.9% sodium chloride injection with chymotrypsin into the tracheostomy tube as ordered to dilute the sputum. Closely monitor whether the wound has bleeding, and whether there is subcutaneous emphysema around the tracheal incision and chest (manifesting as crepitus or crackling sensation). Cover the tracheal cuff with a layer of wet gauze to moisten the airway. Secure tracheostomy tube with one finger's width clearance between ties and neck. Clean the inner cannula four times daily (adjust frequency based on clinical status). Master emergency protocols for tube dislodgement or obstruction.

(III) Health education

1. Psychological care

Create a warm, comfortable and safe environment. Maintain an enthusiastic, sincere and positive attitude while respecting and understanding the patient. Allow emotional expression and engage family/social support systems by encouraging frequent companionship and emotional support from relatives. Additionally, share some successful treatment cases, or arrange peer testimonials to strengthen therapeutic confidence.

2. Dietary guidance

Advise patients to consume high-calorie, high-protein, vitamin-rich and fiber-rich semi-liquid or liquid diets that are easily digestible, and avoid rough, dry, hard, thorny, spicy and other irritating foods.

3. Positioning instruction

Educate patients on the critical importance of posture modification and breathing techniques for improving respiratory function.

4. Tracheostomy management

One week pre-discharge, train patients and their families to clean the tracheal tube. Pay attention to the respiratory status, incision, and tracheal bleeding. Secure the tracheostomy tube with one finger's width clearance between ties and neck to prevent dislodgement. Guide patients to cover the tracheal tube with two layers of gauze, and be careful not to cover the tube opening with quilts, clothing, or paper towels to prevent breathing from being affected and foreign objects from entering the trachea.

5. Communication and guidance

Guide patients to use writing boards, pen and paper, language functions on smartphones, etc., for verbal communication. Patients with low education or visual and hearing impairments can use other tools or be taught simple sign language.

6. Others

Maintain warmth, minimize exposure to crowded areas as much as possible. Balance activity and rest and strictly prohibit showers/swimming.

9. Malignant pleural effusion

Malignant pleural effusion refers to the accumulation of fluid within the pleural cavity caused by metastatic involvement of the pleura or primary pleural tumors. This condition represents a clinical manifestation in patients with advanced-stage malignancies.

(I) Clinical manifestations

Most patients exhibit cachexia characteristics typical of advanced cancer, including weight loss, emaciation, fatigue, anemia, etc. Patients typically present with progressively worsening dyspnea, pleuritic pain, and cough.

(II) Nursing

1. Routine care

(1) Rest and positioning: Maintain bed rest to reduce oxygen consumption and alleviate dyspnea. Depending on the location of the pleural effusion, patients generally take a semi-recumbent position or a side-lying position to reduce the pressure of the pleural effusion on the healthy lung. After fluid resolution, continue convalescence for 2–3 months with strict fatigue avoidance.

(2) Oxygen therapy: Administer nasal cannula oxygen according to dyspnea severity and clinical status, progressing to mask oxygenation if necessary. This improves hypoxia while reducing oxygen demand.

(3) Nutritional support: Provide high-energy, high-protein, vitamin-rich and easily digestible foods to enhance immune resistance.

(4) Psychological support: Reassure patients and families through active emotional observation and attentive listening. Deliver timely psychological guidance while teaching relaxation techniques to mitigate fear and build therapeutic confidence.

After the body temperature returns to normal and the pleural fluid is aspirated or absorbed and the condition permits, patients are encouraged to gradually get out of bed and move around to increase vital capacity.

2. Condition assessment and monitoring

(1) Assessment: (i) Assess the severity and character of cough, expectoration, and dyspnea. (ii) Assess for pleuritic pain – specifically its

location and nature. (iii) Monitor vital signs and arterial blood gas indicators. (iv) Examine chest signs, such as dullness to percussion and whether breath sounds are clear. (v) Assess whether patients with malignant pleural effusion are accompanied by weight loss, anemia, cachexia, and supraclavicular lymphadenopathy. (vi) Assess patients' psychological state.

(2) Observation: (i) Continuously observe the patient's pleuritic pain intensity, dyspnea severity, and vital sign trends, with particular attention to temperature fluctuations. (ii) Monitor changes in blood oxygen saturation or arterial blood gas analysis. (iii) For post-thoracentesis patients: Closely observe changes in breathing, pulse, and blood pressure, and pay attention to whether there is bleeding or fluid seepage at the puncture site.

(III) Health education

1. Maintaining catheter patency

According to the amount and nature of the pleural effusion, intermittent open drainage should be performed as directed by doctors to avoid a sudden drop in blood pressure caused by rapid drainage.

2. Catheter securement

Use the SM patch to stick the external part of the catheter to the chest and abdomen in order, pay attention to the degree of sticking, and replace it immediately if it becomes loose. Patients should maintain bed rest to minimize catheter tension.

3. Dietary guidance

Repeated chest extraction will consume too much energy for the body and cause a large amount of protein loss. Nutrition should be strengthened. It is advisable to eat high-protein, high-vitamin, high-calorie, easily digestible foods, and avoid dry and hard foods, in order to enhance the body's resistance.

4. Psychological support

Create a warm, comfortable and safe environment. Demonstrate warmth, sincerity, and positivity while respecting and validating the patient's emotions. At the same time, coach patients in maintaining emotional equilibrium and permit therapeutic emotional expression. Give full play to their family and social support systems, and encourage their relatives and friends to accompany, support and care for them to enhance their confidence in treatment.

5. Follow-up

Instruct patients to take medication as directed by their doctors, undergo regular checkups, and go to the hospital immediately for treatment if chest pain or difficulty breathing occurs.

6. Posture guidance

Instruct patients to rest in the affected side-lying or semi-recumbent position, and emphasize the critical importance of posture modification and breathing techniques to improve respiratory function and alleviate pain.

7. Rest and activity

Keep the indoor environment clean, quiet and tidy. Avoid fatigue, prone position and excessive bending to prevent the catheter from being bent and causing pericardial injury or poor drainage. Enforce bed rest, adopting the affected-side position for chest pain and semi-Fowler's for dyspnea. After the symptoms are relieved, patients can do some activities appropriately and avoid fatigue or a cold.

8. Medication instructions

Monitor drug efficacy and adverse reactions, timely detect changes in patients' conditions and treat them symptomatically. Regularly monitor blood routine, liver and kidney function, etc.

9. Daily living instructions

(1) Ensure adequate sleep, avoid fatigue, and emotional excitement. Adjust clothing with temperature changes to avoid respiratory infections.

(2) Strictly abstain from tobacco and alcohol while maintaining nutritional intake.

(3) Pay attention to personal hygiene. Strict prohibition of spitting in public. When coughing or sneezing, cover the mouth and nose with a tissue. Wear a mask when going out.

(4) Keep rooms bright, dry and well ventilated. Even in winter, it should

be ventilated twice a day for 30 minutes each time.

10. Malignant pericardial effusion

Malignant pericardial effusion refers to the excessive accumulation of fluid in the pericardial cavity caused by malignant tumors. It is one of the common complications in patients with advanced cancer.

(I) Clinical manifestations

Primary clinical features include dyspnea, palpitations, hepatosplenomegaly, etc.

(II) Nursing

Patients with acute cardiac tamponade may experience profuse sweating, restlessness, and decreased blood pressure. Pericardiocentesis should be performed as soon as possible as a life-saving measure.

1. Fluid drainage care

Strictly prohibit showers for 48 hours post-catheter insertion/removal to prevent site moisture. Carefully observe the wound for exudate. If there is exudate, change the dressing immediately to prevent infection.

(1) Monitor respiration rate, heart rate, blood pressure, and complexion, and record the properties, color, and amount of drainage fluid.

(2) Enforce absolute bed rest for 4 hours after surgery. Assess heart rate, pulse, blood pressure, and respiration every 30 minutes until hemodynamic

stability is achieved.

2. Medical care

(1) Position patients in a forward-leaning or semi-Fowler's position for rest; for severe respiratory distress, use an orthopneic position (sitting upright).

(2) Administer supplemental oxygen via nasal cannula at 3 L/min or switch to mask oxygenation if clinically indicated.

(3) Continuously assess patient comfort levels and promptly detect changes in their condition.

(4) Simultaneously monitor respiratory rate, rhythm and depth, heart rate, and blood pressure changes.

(5) Accurately record intake and output, daily weights, and pay attention to whether there is edema in the sagging parts of the body.

(6) During semi-fowler's positioning, pay attention to the sacrum, inner and outer ankles, heels, etc., to prevent the occurrence of pressure sores.

3. Nutritional care

Malignant tumors increase metabolic consumption. Pericardial effusion is mainly composed of fibrin and cells, which causes protein loss during the extraction process. Provide high-protein, high-calorie, and easily digestible food. Reduce intake of gas-producing foods such as milk to prevent bowel distension and diaphragmatic elevation. Low-salt foods are the main ones, and salt-free foods should be chosen if edema is severe.

4. Psychological support

Reassure patients and families through active emotional observation and attentive listening. Deliver timely psychological guidance while teaching relaxation techniques to mitigate fear and build therapeutic confidence.

5. Take breaks

Strengthen basic nursing care, keep the ward clean, bright and quiet. After pericardiocentesis, enforce absolute bed rest and minimize movement.

6. Cough management

Patients with a cough can be given nebulized inhalation as prescribed by doctors to dilute the sputum. If accompanied by a severe cough, codeine can be taken orally.

(III) Health education

1. Maintaining catheter patency

Open drainage intermittently based on pericardial effusion volume and characteristics, typically 2-6 times daily for 30-60 minutes per session. After drainage completion, instill prescribed medications into the pericardial cavity via the catheter. Following medication administration, flush the lumen with 2-4mL heparinized saline (12.5-25 U/mL concentration) to prevent occlusion.

2. Catheter securement

Use the SM patch to stick the external part of the catheter to the chest and abdomen in order, pay attention to the degree of sticking, and replace it immediately if it becomes loose. Patients should maintain bed rest to minimize catheter tension.

3. Dietary guidance

Consume primarily soft, easily digestible foods that are high in calories, protein, vitamins and fiber. Avoid dry and hard food.

4. Psychological support

Create a warm, comfortable and safe environment. Demonstrate warmth, sincerity, and positivity while respecting and validating the patient's emotions. At the same time, coach patients in maintaining emotional equilibrium and permit therapeutic emotional expression. Give full play to their family and social support systems, and encourage their relatives and friends to accompany, support and care for them to enhance their confidence in treatment.

5. Follow-up

Instruct patients that if they experience symptoms such as dyspnea, palpitations, cyanosis, cough, etc., and general treatment is ineffective, they should return to the hospital as soon as possible for treatment and regular check-ups.

6. Positioning instruction

Adopt a forward-leaning or semi-Fowler's position for rest. For severe respiratory compromise, use an orthopneic position (upright sitting).

7. Take breaks

Keep the indoor environment clean, quiet and tidy. Avoid fatigue, prone position and excessive bending to prevent the catheter from bending and causing pericardial injury or poor drainage.

11. Malignant peritoneal effusion

Malignant peritoneal effusion refers to pathological fluid accumulation in the peritoneal cavity caused by malignant tumors, which may result from tumor invasion of the peritoneum or by tumor obstruction of lymphatic vessels or veins. It is a common complication in patients with advanced tumors.

(I) Clinical manifestations

Clinical manifestations may include abdominal distension, foot edema, fatigue, shortness of breath, weight loss, and increased abdominal circumference.

(II) Nursing

Malignant ascites represents a severe and frequent complication in advanced malignant tumors.

1. Nutritional management

(1) The primary objectives are to alleviate discomfort and prevent/manage complications.

(2) Diversify the diet, provide high-vitamin, high-protein, low-fat, low-salt, easily digestible diets. Provide a low-salt (3-5 g daily salt intake) or salt-restricted (2 g daily salt intake) diet according to the condition of ascites. The purpose of a low-salt diet is to reduce the retention of water and sodium in the body. Critically, patients with hypoalbuminemia- induced ascites require strict sodium/fluid restriction alongside prescribed albumin infusions. Additionally, strictly avoid irritants and alcohol.

(3) Prioritize lean meat, fish, poultry, and dairy products, limit water and sodium intake. Restrict fluid intake to 1000 mL/day and sodium salt intake to 500-1000 mg/day.

2. Psychological support

Patients with malignant tumor ascites are prone to pessimism and disappointment due to poor prognosis. Provide compassionate support through active listening and disease-specific education to alleviate anxieties and build therapeutic confidence. In view of patients' psychological barriers such as pessimism, despair, anxiety, and depression, patiently explain the importance of intraperitoneal chemotherapy. Help patients accept potential treatment-related discomforts while reassuring them through prompt management of adverse reactions to ensure treatment compliance.

3. Activity and rest

Patients need to be provided with a comfortable and clean recuperation environment, with adequate rest and activities. Guide patients in graded activity based on clinical status, ensuring exertion never exceeds tolerance thresholds. Patients with a large amount of ascites should strictly follow bed rest and take a semi-recumbent position to move the diaphragm downward and alleviate breathing difficulties.

4. Basic care

Because patients' abdomen is swollen, with the abdominal wall taut and shiny, and the skin thin and easily scratched, maintain skin cleanliness and dryness using tepid water sponging. Wear loose cotton clothes, and change clothes and bedding in time if dampened. Use sponge pads on the pressure parts. Reposition patient q2h with gentle massage to prevent pressure injuries. Pay attention to bowel movements, and for those with constipation due to long-term bed rest, laxatives such as lactulose can be given to relieve symptoms if necessary.

(III) Health education

1. Maintaining catheter patency

Open drainage intermittently based on ascites volume/characteristics as prescribed, preventing rapid drainage that may cause abrupt hypotension.

2. Catheter securement

Pay attention to the adhesive integrity and replace it immediately if loose. Maintain bed rest to minimize catheter tension.

3. Dietary guidance

Consume primarily soft, easily digestible foods that are high-calorie, high-protein, low-fat, low-sodium, and vitamin-fiber rich. Strictly avoid dry/hard foods.

4. Psychological support

Create a warm, comfortable and safe environment. Demonstrate warmth, sincerity, and positivity while respecting and validating the patient's emotions. At the same time, coach patients in maintaining emotional equilibrium and permit therapeutic emotional expression. Give full play to their family and social support systems, and encourage their relatives and friends to accompany, support and care for them more, so as to enhance their confidence in treatment.

5. Follow-up

Instruct patients that if they experience symptoms such as abdominal distension, increased abdominal circumference, shortness of breath, foot edema, oliguria, and weight loss, and general treatment is ineffective, they should return to the hospital as soon as possible for treatment and regular checkups.

6. Positioning instruction

Adopt a forward-leaning or semi-Fowler's position for rest. For severe respiratory compromise, use an orthopneic position (upright sitting).

7. Take breaks

Keep the indoor environment clean, quiet and tidy. Avoid fatigue, prone position and excessive bending to prevent the catheter from bending and causing pericardial injury or poor drainage.

8. Disease education

Train patients and their families to master the basic knowledge of the disease and eliminate various inducements. Guide patients on how to take care of themselves, maintain health after discharge and sustain long-term care plan adherence. Educate patients and their family carefully monitor for critical symptoms (diarrhea, abdominal distension, oliguria, leg edema) requiring urgent care, to keep physical condition at a good level.